The *On Becoming* Series

On Becoming Birthwise

On Becoming Babywise

On Becoming Babywise II

On Becoming Pretoddlerwise

On Becoming Toddlerwise

On Becoming Pottywise for Toddlers

On Becoming Preschoolwise

On Becoming Childwise

On Becoming Preteenwise

On Becoming Teenwise

What Healthcare Professionals Say About *On Becoming Babywise*

My introduction to *On Becoming Babywise* came over 20 years ago when a discerning member in my practice noticed my frustration with the growing numbers of fatigued mothers, fussy babies and their sleepless nights. I was handed a set of audio tapes of this series. Being profoundly impressed with the insightfulness and relevance of the content, I began applying the principles in my practice. The change was dramatic, as I watched the incidence of colicky babies, sleep-disturbed and frustrated parents drop precipitously. Word of mouth among our community has helped our practice grow exponentially. I cannot imagine any pediatrician that has come in contact with this resource not making it part of their practice.

Jim Pearson, M.D.
Johnson City, Tennessee

As family physicians and a husband-wife team, we are often asked questions related to parenting and the general care of children. Most of our basic responses are found in *On Becoming Babywise*. For answering parenting questions, it has become a practical guide, giving us a sense of competence and confidence as physicians and as parents. When the principles are put into practice, parents reap abundant rewards.

Tony Burden, M.D., and Margaret Burden, M.D.
Bellingham, Washington

Babywise provides sound parenting advice and common sense pediatric care to many parents who are confused, frustrated, and downright sleep deprived. As a pediatrician and father of four, my wife and I routinely receive positive feedback regarding our children's behavior and sleep habits. Parents feel confident and relaxed when they have a plan and a goal for their infant and family. Once a family has found success with the principles in *Babywise*, they pass along their satisfaction to every new parent they meet. Simply put, "It works!"

David M. Miller, M.D.
Superior, Colorado

I am a practicing pediatrician and assistant professor of pediatrics. Residents and new mothers I work with have found *On Becoming Babywise* overwhelmingly successful. My residents report a positive difference in the confidence of new mothers who work with this plan compared to those who do not. The freedom *Babywise* provides a new mother is so refreshing. Life is predictable, allowing her to be proactive in parenting, not reactive, which usually produces less-than-desirable results. My parents become baby-wise with *Babywise*.

Linda Meloy, M.D.
Richmond, Virginia

As a pediatrician, I cannot argue with the success of *On Becoming Babywise*. It is such a practical approach to parenting. It provides infants with needed structure and stability and brings the joy and love so needed in our homes today. The effects of not using *On Becoming Babywise* show up very quickly. That is why I have made these principles a priority of discussion in every well-child care visit. Parents constantly tell me, "It changed our lives."

Janet Dunn, M.D.
Bellefontaine, Ohio

As a practicing pediatrician, husband, and father, I enthusiastically recommend *On Becoming Babywise*. I found the principles contained within to be a sigh of welcome relief to sleepless, weary parents, and more than an ounce of prevention for those who adopt these concepts from the start. I am convinced that the well-tested principles of *Babywise* produce confident parents, secure and content infants, and peaceful and orderly homes.

David Blank, M.D.
Longmont, Colorado

As an obstetrician and a mother, my concern for a healthy outcome continues beyond the moment of delivery. Because the principles of *On Becoming Babywise* are so effective, I consider it part of my extended health care for the entire family. The principles are simple, yet amazing. They consistently produce babies who are healthy, content, and who sleep through the night at an early age. Feeding a baby on demand simply cannot compare to the overall healthy benefits of *Babywise*. The concepts take the guesswork out of early parenting and provide new moms the confidence of knowing what happens next. Not following the principles of *Babywise* is a potential health concern.

Sharon Nelson, M.D.
Glendale, California

Medical school in no way prepared me for one of the more demanding aspects of my practice: dealing with infant feeding. The theory of feeding a baby whenever it cries, which was standard teaching, was not only without justification—it simply did not meet the needs of my patients. Since being introduced to the principles of *On Becoming Babywise*, I have been convinced of its effectiveness in establishing sleep patterns and in decreasing the frequency of problems associated with infant feeding. If thriving children and happy, rested parents were not enough, my greatest commendation of *On Becoming Babywise* is that my own children are being raised by these precepts.

Craig Lloyd, M.D.
Brisbane, Australia

As a Mom, I parented both ways. As a certified lactation educator, I know how discouraging it is to feed a baby around the clock with no apparent advantage and how fatigue will affect her milk supply. I also know how discouraging the first eighteen months of parenting can be without a plan. I know, because with my first child, I did everything the opposite of what is taught in this book. Before my second baby was born, I was introduced to the *Babywise* concepts. Applying the principles revolutionized my thinking. Instead of being in baby bondage, I was liberated to be the mother God wanted me to be. I have consistently used this series with the women I counsel. These mothers have met with tremendous success, whether bottle or breastfeeding.

Barbara Phillips, R.N., C.L.E.
Los Angeles, California

What Moms and Dads Are Saying About *On Becoming Babywise*

After a fatiguing and depressing three months of parenting, my sister-in-law handed me a copy of *Babywise*. It saved my life! Before *Babywise*, I sought help everywhere: books, friends, experienced mothers, even my baby's pediatrician. I received plenty of advice, but no real solutions that could turn around a 24/7 fussy baby. Seven days after applying the *Babywise* principles, my baby was sleeping 9 hours at night, napping during the day, and his fussiness was isolated to an hour in the late afternoon. The amount of common sense wrapped up in this one book is amazing and very definitely life changing.

A mother from West Covina, California

My husband and I had heard all sorts of horror stories and felt so discouraged and defeated before our baby came. Feeding around the clock, unexplained fussiness, and household chaos was not what we wanted. We were sure there had to be a more sane way to parent than that. We were introduced to the *Babywise* concepts a week before our son was born. How timely! As predicted, our happy, contented baby was sleeping through the night at eight weeks. We so appreciate Dr. Bucknam and Mr. Ezzo's insights, and thank them for giving us the confidence to do what is best for our son.

A mother from Denver, Colorado

Without reservation I would recommend this program to anyone—because it works. I demand-fed my first three children, not knowing there was another way. I did not get a complete night's sleep in five years. When friends began to share your principles, I refused to listen to what I thought was simplistic nonsense. I hold a master's degree in early childhood education, and your concepts challenged everything I had been taught.

When our friends' first child slept through the night at six weeks, I was enraged. My husband and I watched as their second and third followed the same pattern. They had everything under control, and so few of the problems that we experienced. When I discovered that I was expecting baby number four, I was depressed for months. The only thing I could focus on was the misery of more sleepless nights and demanding children.

I am ashamed to say that it was out of desperation that we applied your parent-directed feeding concepts. I was humbled. Our baby slept through the night at seven weeks. We could not believe it was that easy. He was a delight, happy and content, something never experienced with the first three. Since then, a fifth child has arrived and, again, success. *On Becoming Babywise* has saved our marriage and family. Thank you.

A mother from Philadelphia, Pennsylvania

My husband and I want to thank you for getting us on the right track from the beginning. It was not easy, because all our friends followed the demand-feeding philosophy and said a schedule was bad for the baby. For these families, children were a major interruption. That did not make sense to us. We stayed with your program, and our baby slept 8 hours through the night at six weeks, and 11 hours at twelve weeks—just like your book says. My friends said exactly what you predicted: that we were lucky and had an easy baby. But we know otherwise. Thank you for being a source of encouragement.

A mother from Fort Worth, Texas

I was at church holding a crying baby, and everyone asked what was wrong with my son. They said they had never before heard him cry. Then they realized, I was holding someone else's baby. Thank you for *On Becoming Babywise*. My wife and I have a happy, contented baby. Before our son was born, we heard so many disturbing stories. My sister had not been out with her husband for three years after the birth of their first son. She went to a mothers' support group but only found other mothers to cry with. No, thank you! Not for my wife. We follow the principles of *PDF*. Because our lives are so predictable, and our son responds so well to routine, we had our first date night after three weeks and once a week ever since. Thank you for helping to keep our family a family.

A father from Tacoma, Washington

Our daughter will be one year old at the end of this month, and

I must tell you that I truly and profoundly enjoyed the first year of her life. A big part of the reason is because we followed the principles of *On Becoming Babywise*. It was not only helpful with my daughter, but it also helped me understand my frustrations with my firstborn! I kept wondering why he was so demanding. Why would he never sleep at night or take decent naps?

I had nursed my son as often as he needed (so I thought)—anytime and anywhere, day and night—until he was 22 months old. And I gave him attention, both quality and quantity. He slept with us at night, but after a few weeks, the baby slept with only me; my husband was sleeping on the couch. I stayed home, gave him a good learning environment, and cooked all natural foods. I did everything the "experts" said to do. But they were so wrong. In the end, it was all for nothing. The only thing I succeeded in doing was to raise a demanding, out-of-control toddler who is not pleasant to be with.

I do not share this to burden you, but to encourage you. Please get the *Babywise* principles out to young families of our nation (Canada) and yours, so they will not have to suffer what we did. Thank you for your sensible teaching.

A mother from Vancouver, British Columbia

My wife and I were introduced to your program while in marriage counseling. It was then that we discovered the trap of child-centered parenting. In the name of "good parenthood," we gave up our marriage—figuratively and nearly literally. We did this for the "baby's good." That sounded sacrificial and was something I wanted to do as a father. But I never realized how faulty that thinking was until I read your first two chapters. Your book makes sense out of nonsense.

After 18 months of misery, we started our son on a routine. After four nights he began sleeping through the night, and my wife began to sleep with me—but this time alone. What a difference a good night's sleep makes to a toddler's disposition! We had a new son. Get these vital principles out to every family of childbearing age.

A father from Atlanta, Georgia

ON BECOMING BABY WISE

Giving Your Infant the *GIFT* of Nighttime Sleep

ROBERT BUCKNAM, M.D.
GARY EZZO, M.A.

ON BECOMING BABYWISE®

Giving Your Infant the GIFT of Nighttime Sleep

Join us online
www.Facebook/Babywise.Life

Published in Partnership with
Hawksflight & Associates/Charleston Publishing Group, Inc

ISBN: 978-1-932740-53-0
Printed in the United States of America

Charleston Publishing Group, Inc
Administrative Office
2160 Cheswick Lane
Mount Pleasant, SC 29466

Print Run/Year
113 / 23

Dedicated to:

Ashley Nicole
The first to call us Grammie and Grandpa

ACKNOWLEDGMENTS

According to a host of online dictionaries, the purpose of an "acknowledgment" is to express a debt of gratitude and appreciation to someone who otherwise would not be recognized. These pages exist for that reason. While the cover of this book displays our names as Authors, in truth there were many people from within our community of thought who applied their time, energy and giftedness to help make this book a joint venture for the common good. Most readers will never personally meet these behind-the-scene individuals, but each reader will be the benefactor of their labor.

Where would we be without our medical advisors and friends? We especially wish to thank Dr. Robert Turner for providing oversight with matters pertaining to pediatric neurology and Doctors Jim Pearson, Stuart Eldridge and Luke Nightingale, who never grew weary with our many questions. And special thanks to our long-time friends, Dr. Eleanor and Mr. Clay Womack for their contribution in Chapter Ten related to parenting twins and triplets.

We also wish to express our deep gratitude and appreciation to Nathan Babcock for his editorial review. The combination of his intellect and passion for clarity came at a critical intersection of this update. Joining Nathan are Tommye Gadol and Geoff and Alicia Bongers, whose helpful insights and comments were highly prized and greatly appreciated. We also acknowledge the assistance of Cyndi Bird who routinely provided us numerous examples and insights related to nap and waketime challenges encountered by the Moms under her watchful eye. There are also Joe and Nancy Barlow whose constant encouragement and support have no limits.

Turning our appreciation closer to home, we are honored

to serve with a team of young couples whose collective voices brought a level of clarity to the message that we alone could have never achieved. Among the many are Rich and Julie Young who played an integral role in refining many of the *Babywise* concepts. Joining the Young's are Greg and Tara Banks, Alan and Candace Furness, and Shawn and Connie Wood and Linda Gage. To all our contributors, we say, "Thank you."

Contents

Foreword

After completing medical school and serving my residency in obstetrics and gynecology, I felt knowledgeable enough to be a parent. Between my wife's degree in child development and my medical training, how hard could this parenting thing be? We would just do what comes naturally and follow our instincts. Right? Wrong!

Soon after the birth of our first son, we quickly found our enthusiasm and confidence turned into exhaustion and frustration. My wife was up four times at night, and my son was excessively fussy during the day. The unsolicited advice typically offered by colleagues was to feed more often since it was assumed my son cried because he was hungry. We did feed him, around the clock, every two hours. As we found out later, that was the cause of the problem, not the cure.

Scientists can put a man on the moon, but they cannot answer the most basic problems of early parenting: how to have a happy and contented baby who sleeps continually through the night like the rest of the family and a mother who is not in a perpetual state of exhaustion.

Through our common interest in children and parenting, my wife and I became acquainted with the work and accomplishments of Gary and Anne Marie Ezzo. The Ezzos' basic and loving concepts for nurturing newborns virtually eliminated the problems listed above and many more. I have personally observed infants who were guided by the Ezzos' principles and those who were not. It became obvious that parents equipped with the right information do make a difference.

That was one reason why, nearly 30 years ago, I made the transition from obstetrics to pediatrics and with the switch came the medically sound principles of *Babywise*. They work consistently, not only for millions of children already touched by the work of Gary and Anne Marie, but also for my four children, my colleagues' children, my friends' children, and all my patients.

To say the least, *Babywise* has brought a needed reformation to pediatric counsel given to new parents. When parents come in looking exhausted and discouraged and tell me their woeful stories of sleepless nights and fussy babies, I can give them a positive prescription that cures the problem—I hand them *On Becoming Babywise*.

Robert Bucknam, MD
Louisville, Colorado

Introduction

The principles of *Babywise* were first shared in 1984. Sarah was the first baby girl raised with the principles; Kenny was the first boy. Both thrived on mother's milk and a basic routine, and both slept through the night by seven weeks. It was that easy. From friend to friend, city to city, state to state, and country to country, the positive message continues to spread. Today we no longer count the success stories in thousands or even in tens of thousands, but in millions of happy, healthy babies who were given the *gift* of nighttime sleep.

As with the previous editions, this update does not provide parents a list of *do's* and *don'ts*. We wish parenting were that easy. Rather, our larger objective is to help prepare minds for the incredible task of raising a child. We believe the preparation of the mind is far more important than the preparation of the nursery. Your baby will not care if his head rests on designer sheets or beside Disney characters, nor is your success tied to his wardrobe or bedroom accessories, but rather to the beliefs and convictions that will eventually shape your parenting experience.

It is our opinion that the achievements of healthy growth, contented babies, good naps, and playful waketimes, as well as the gift of nighttime sleep, are too valuable to be left to chance. They need to be parent-directed and parent-managed. These are attainable conclusions, because infants are born with the *capacity* to achieve these outcomes and, equally important, the *need* to achieve them. Our goal is to demonstrate *how* this is done, but only after we explain *why* it should be done.

We realize there are a number of parenting theories being marketed today, most of which come gift-wrapped with unrealistic promises and unnecessary burdens. In light of the many options, how can new parents know what approach is best for their families? Since every philosophy of parenting has a corresponding outcome unique to that philosophy, we encourage new and expectant parents to consider, evaluate, and decide which approach is best for their families. This can be accomplished by observing the end results. Spend time with relatives and friends who follow the La Leche League/Attachment Parenting style of infant care. Observe those who practice hyperscheduling, and certainly evaluate the outcomes associated with *Babywise.*

In which homes do you observe order, peace, and tranquility? Consider the marriages as well as the children. Is Mom in a perpetual state of exhaustion? Is she nursing every two hours or less? Is Dad sleeping on the couch? What is family life like when a child is 6, 12 and 18 months old? Is Mom stressed, frustrated, or lacking confidence? Is the baby stressed, exhausted or insecure? When the baby is nine months old, can the parents leave the room without the baby falling apart emotionally? We believe the best evaluation of any parenting philosophy, including the one found in this book, is not found in the reasoning or the logic of the hypothesis but in the end results. Let your eyes confirm what works and what does not. You will be most confident in your parenting when you see the desired results lived out in other families using the same approach. Look at the *fruit* and then trace it back to its *seed* source.

The Appendices section of this book contains charts, worksheets, and additional information relating to infant care. Appendices of a book should never be considered less important than the general reading, but only of *different* importance. Please read them in the order in which they are referred to in the chapters.

There are some matters of terminology that we would like to

address. When you read through each chapter, you will see that we predominantly used the masculine gender in our illustrations. This was done for our convenience. The principles will, of course, work equally well with girls. Also, in our attempt to speak directly to our community of parents, we often use the pronouns *you*, *your*, and *yours* to address our readers. While we realize that not everyone reading this book is a parent, the vast majority are, thus we toggled between second and third-person expressions. Finally, the name of the child most often referred to in this book is "Baby."

The principles contained within these pages can help parents develop workable strategies that meet the needs of their babies and the rest of the family. These have worked for millions of parents, and when faithfully applied can work wonderfully for you! However, your pediatrician or family practitioner should always be consulted when questions arise about the health and welfare of your baby.

Finally, connect with new and experienced *Babywise* moms at *www.Facebook.com/BabywiseLife*. There you will find additional resources, encouragement and answers to your parenting questions.

Enjoy the journey!

Gary Ezzo

Chapter One
Right Beginnings

Apart from the orphaned child, most people grow up in families in which from birth onward, they learn a way of life that gives meaning to their very existence. For most of us, the word *home* carries more than just casual memories of a time and place where we spent our childhood; it was the first society from which we learned about life itself. It is within the confines of home that everyone first experiences the repertoire of human emotions and observes how others respond. We learn the meaning of sympathy, empathy, and caring. We absorb family and cultural values, and measure our commitment to those values by how others respond to them. The home is where love is first defined by the care and attention we receive and becomes the place where security is gained, lost, or possibly, never obtained.

The word *home* is so laden with significance that one cannot begin a conversation about baby care without first speaking to the persuasive influence that the home environment exerts, especially during the critical first year. From the first breath to the last day on earth, nothing will impact a person's life more than the influence a mom and dad bring to the home environment. That is because no other relationship in a child's life has greater and more lasting significance than that between parent and child. In the same way, no other relationship can test one's personality and resolve more than children can with their parents.

What are the basic concerns of parenthood? What questions should expectant couples be asking, and what assumptions should they be embracing or shedding, when it comes to preparing themselves for the lifelong commitment of parenthood?

While we realize that parenting is very personal, we also know there are certain assumptions about babies and baby care that can serve as powerful guides to achieve successful outcomes. Just as true, however, there are some assumptions, we unashamedly will tell you to avoid if you are seeking to secure for your baby a firm physical, emotional and neurologic foundation on which to build.

The Challenge

All too often, couples enter parenting hoping that an all-knowing sense of clarity will spontaneously emerge without having to put effort into learning parenting basics. Even with some classroom preparation, first-time parents are often shocked once the baby arrives by how much their lives change to accommodate the needs of their newborn. For Mom, the challenge is physical and emotional. She can no longer rely on the in-utero relationship that took care of protecting and nurturing her baby. Now specific infant needs must be matched with understanding of how to best satisfy those needs. It is a time when she becomes acquainted with all the new baby sounds that will suddenly trigger a variety of emotions never previously experienced. She will be struck by the compelling sensation to nurture, protect, and provide for her baby.

It is also an adjustment time for Dad, starting with a need to share his best friend, his wife, with his son or daughter. In essence he is giving up something to gain more. Change also impacts Mom and Dad's free time. The times spent together before Baby arrived needed less planning; but now, nothing can be done spur of the moment without first asking, "What about the baby?" With a newborn in the home, life changes forever, and expectant parents should fully embrace what will become the *new normal*. However, this is where the challenge comes in.

Some parents assume optimistically that life will not change drastically with a newborn in the home. That is not true, but neither is the opposite extreme that expects the tranquility of pre-baby home life to dissolve into a hopeless state of on-going chaos. With a baby in your near future, life as you know it will change, for change is the reality of the day. How successfully parents navigate and manage those changes is dependent on their understanding of the micro and macro needs that all babies share—and, of course, the best way to meet those needs.

WHAT'S MISSING?

We have counseled many couples that started their journey in parenting with high hopes and the best intentions to love and nurture their newborn, only to see their dreams reduced to a nightmare of survival. Who are these people? They are parents like so many others: the sweet couple you met in your birthing class, the family down the street, or the next-door neighbor with the cute wooden stork on the front lawn wrapped with pink balloons announcing the birth of Alexis. These mothers and fathers are equipped with a long list of baby facts, but they often lack *understanding* of how all those facts fit together in the big picture of life. While facts can provide a plan, only understanding can provide the purpose. What is understanding, and why is it important?

Understanding, as a concept of learning, is the mechanism that gives meaning and value to facts. It reaches beyond the moment and looks into the future. Parenting with purposeful understanding connects each moment with a day, a day with a week, a week with a month, and a month of doing with a year of accomplishments. Understanding allows parents to find the right course and stay there with a minimal number of course corrections. It is also a prerequisite necessary for making wise and productive decisions. Our goal in this book is to provide new and expectant parents with the type of understanding that yields confidence for Mom and Dad, and an abiding security for their baby.

START HERE: BUILDING A LOVING HOME ENVIRONMENT

With 30 years of pediatric and parent-coaching experience behind us, along with several million adherents to the *Babywise* principles, we have learned a few things about newborns, parents, and parenting philosophies. At the top of the list is this truth: The outcomes common to *Babywise* infants are developmental achievements too valuable to be left to chance. They are parent-directed and not child-led.

Second, we know that parents naturally and instantly fall in love with their babies. That is the way of parental love. However, falling in love with your baby is not the same thing as providing your baby a loving home environment. A healthy home environment starts with Mom and Dad's commitment to each other, from which a more perfect love is communicated to their children.

Third, a loving home environment is not something that naturally emerges. It takes work and sacrifice, and it requires that both Mom and Dad be intentional in their love for each other. It also requires parents to gain understanding of the three prevailing influences that shape every child's destiny. The first is his genetic disposition inherited from Mom and Dad. This speaks to a baby's physical and intellectual potential. The second great influence comes through his temperament, which is that dimension of his personality governing whether he is outgoing, shy, funny, or even keel. The third great influence is the home environment created by Mom and Dad.

While parents cannot change their child's genetic inscription or their child's temperament, they will influence the home environment and thus shape their child's destiny. What defines the home environment? This is where children first learn of love. From whom will they learn it? In part, they will learn from Mom, and in part from Dad, but most persuasively from Mom and Dad working as a team. This is because a mother and father cannot communicate the total message of love apart from the oneness that was formed in the bonds of their own marriage.

Marriage is more than a legal status between two people; it is a living entity that reflects a special bond between a man and a woman—it is a unique relationship, one without parallel. While marriage transcends all other relationships, it is not disconnected from parenting. Just as the human heart pumps oxygen-rich blood to the body, so a healthy marriage fuels all the cells that make parenting come alive. It is truly an amazing relationship! That is why couples with great marriages make great parents, and their children are the benefactors.

THE MARRIAGE FACTOR

The fairy-tale conclusion, "and they lived happily ever after," assumes happiness is an effortless, spontaneous outcome of marriage. This is far from being true. Men are not born good husbands, nor women good wives. They become that way only through self-sacrifice, patience, and a devotional commitment to the happiness and welfare of the other.

It, therefore, serves a husband and wife to remember that they will not *find* long-term happiness in marriage, but rather they can *achieve* it through marriage, which trickles down to their parenting. This means the husband-wife union is not just a good first step towards successful child-rearing, but it is in fact a necessary one—one on which your children will come to depend.

Although the primary emphasis of this book is nurturing your newborn, we would be remiss in our educational efforts if we failed to explain what turns hope into reality. We believe that if you really love your children, you will give them the gift of love, security, and a sense of belonging that can only be derived from an on-going demonstration of your love for each other as a husband and wife.

A healthy and vibrant marriage relationship is essential to

the emotional health of children (as well as to Mom and Dad's emotional welfare). When there is harmony in the marriage, there is an infused stability within the family. Even more certain, strong marriages provide a haven of security for children as they mature. That is because the "love" message between Mom and Dad, creates a sense of certainty for children. When a child observes the special friendship and emotional togetherness of his parents, he is naturally more secure because of his confidence in Mom and Dad's relationship. Let's dig a little deeper into this.

The Impact on Children

Humans, unlike members of the animal kingdom, possess a particular emotional DNA strand that will not allow the inner person to be truly satisfied with just the physical side of the marriage relationship. That is, in part, what distinguishes us as humans! When a husband and wife are not one with each other in regard to emotional, physical, social oneness, they have gaps in their relationship, which have unintended consequences extending to their children.

While a husband or wife might be able to cope with the missing part, children do not fare as well. Babies are not able to rely on reason or intellect to measure the stability of the world around them, so they intuitively reach out with their senses. We cannot over emphasize this point: the more parents demonstrate love for each other, the more they saturate their child's senses with confidence of a loving, safe and secure world.

Why is this important to understand? Because it has a direct tie to your baby's developing brain! To put it simply, the infant brain, like the adult brain, functions in one of two primary modes. It is either in the "thriving" mode (learning and growing), or it is in the "survival" mode, (coping and protecting.) However, the brain cannot be in both modes at the same time. This is relevant, since the health of a baby's brain is tied to the amount of time it stays in the learning mode.

There is something about the observable love of Mom and Dad's relationship that profoundly shapes the neural-wiring of a young child's brain. It is no wonder that researchers are now reporting that one of the most reliable predictors of a child's future emotional security and cognitive success is not the mother-child "attachment," but what the child observes in the husband-wife attachment.[1]

From early infancy onward, children possess a survival mechanism that intuitively uses Mom and Dad's relationship as the baseline for their overall sense of security and confirmation. If the child is continually sensing marital stability, the baby's brain gravitates toward healthy growth patterns. However, if the child perceives even the slightest threat of marital instability, the brain is forced to take the energy necessary for healthy growth and transfer it into coping and survival strategies.

That marriage relationship provides children with a layer of love and security that cannot be achieved through the direct parent-child relationship—even during the baby years. When you put all of these factors together, they add up to a healthy home environment that allows a baby to thrive.

THE WARNING

Too often, parents lose sight of the bigger picture, or maybe they never understood it. They get lost in a parenting wonderland of photos, footsteps and first words. Baby becomes central to their existence, to the exclusion of their own relationship as a husband and wife. That might be a fun diversion for Mom and Dad for awhile, but it is not helpful to the baby. Thus, the greatest overall influence parents have on their children comes not in their roles as individual parents, but in their shared role as husband and wife.

Think about it. When the marriage relationship is beautiful, what impressionable child would not desire to share in its joy? When two are beautifully *one*, what child would not seek the comforts of their togetherness? Parents define for their children the meaning of love as much by what happens in their relationship as anything they may do for their children. Healthy parenting flows from healthy marriages. Protect and keep yours safe!

MEETING EVERYONE'S NEEDS

What do parents need to know to keep their marriages alive and well so they can maximize their parenting influence? Here are a few action principles:

1. *Continue living! Life does not stop once the baby arrives. It may slow down for a few weeks, but it should not stop entirely.* When a couple becomes a mother and a father, they do not stop being a daughter or son, a brother or sister, or a friend. Relationships important before the baby comes will still be important after the baby arrives. They are worth protecting and keeping. Show hospitality and invite the new grandparents and friends over as soon as life settles down.

2. *Date your spouse.* If you had a weekly date-night before the baby was born, continue that practice as soon as you can after the baby arrives. If you did not have a weekly date-night, now may be a good time to start. It does not have to be an expensive or late evening, but keeping your marriage fresh is the starting point of keeping your entire family emotionally healthy.

3. *Continue those loving gestures that were enjoyed before the baby came along.* If there was a special activity that you enjoyed previously, you should plan it into your schedule. If a Dad brings home a gift for Baby, how about one for Mom as well? The idea here is basic. The loving gestures that marked the marriage relationship as special—before the baby came—need to be kept special throughout the parenting years.

4. *Practice Couch Time.*
At the end of each workday, spend at least 15 minutes sitting with your spouse discussing the day's events. This simple ges-

ture provides children a tangible sense of their parents' togetherness and fulfills one of their greatest emotional needs—the need to know Mom and Dad love for each other. Couch time provides the visual marker that children are looking for. When children connect their intuitive need-to-know their world is safe and secure with the confirmation of Mom and Dad's love relationship, then security is realized and "healthy brain" growth takes place. When children sense harmony in the marriage relationship, there is an infused stability that spreads throughout the entire home.

5. *Know what to expect of each other before your baby arrives.* For new parents, those first several days at home with a new baby are the most difficult, simply because everything is new and unfolding. Every couple seems to naturally find their groove of family responsibility before the baby arrives, but what about after? If this is your first child, you have yet to hear the various little sounds that your baby will make or experience how his cry will impact your postpartum emotions. Add these factors to the feeding and sleep challenges, and you will quickly discover just how stressful the first few weeks can be.

To help minimize the stress a baby can bring into a normal home, parents should take the time to work through their expectations of each other, before their baby is born. Each person should know what household activity or chore he or she will be responsible for. Who will take care of the laundry and meals, shopping, vacuuming, furniture dusting, and who will get up to get the baby for the middle-of-the-night feeding?

This may seem like an insignificant to-do list right now, but we assure you, these common household chores are not so insignificant after the baby arrives. Take some time and review The "Who Will do What" List below. Check the boxes that represent Dad's duties and those belonging to Mom. Keep in mind there will be visiting relatives, so a fair "price of admission" to see the baby is helping around the house.

THE "WHO WILL DO WHAT" LIST

MOM	HOUSEHOLD RESPONSIBILITIES	DAD
☐	Wash laundry	☐
☐	Fold laundry	☐
☐	Put away laundry	☐
☐	Ironing	☐
☐	Dry cleaning drop-off	☐
☐	Dry cleaning pick-up	☐
☐	Grocery shopping	☐
☐	Put away groceries	☐
☐	Prepare meals	☐
☐	Breakfast	☐
☐	Lunch	☐
☐	Dinner	☐
☐	Wash Dishes	☐
☐	Load dishwasher	☐
☐	General home care	☐
☐	Clean bathrooms	☐
☐	Vacuum	☐
☐	Dust	☐
☐	Make bed	☐
☐	Change bed linens	☐
☐	Water plants	☐
☐	Take out trash/recycling	☐
☐	Laundry	☐
☐	Feed pet	☐
☐	Clean up after pet	☐
☐	Walk the dog	☐
☐	Yard work	☐
☐	Get the mail	☐
☐	Pay the bills	☐
☐	Banking	☐
☐	Vehicle maintenance/service	☐
☐	Other ________________	☐

☐	Other ________________	☐
☐	Other ________________	☐
☐	Other ________________	☐

MOM	BABY-CARE RESPONSIBILITY	DAD
☐	Send baby announcements	☐
☐	Write thank-you notes	☐
☐	Feed baby (if bottle fed)	☐
☐	Diaper changes	☐
☐	Get baby at night for feeding	☐
☐	Night Feeding (if bottle fed)	☐
☐	Bathe the baby	☐
☐	Comfort baby at fussy times	☐
☐	Care for other children	☐
☐	Other ________________	☐
☐	Other ________________	☐
☐	Other ________________	☐
☐	Other ________________	☐

A WORD TO THE SINGLE PARENT

Throughout life, we face unexpected challenges that detract from the ideal. In the home environment, the ideal is to operate as a parent from the strength of your marriage. We realize that ideal is not present in every home. The death of a spouse, a divorce or an unplanned pregnancy can cause our dreams to disappear under a cloud of discouragement. Having worked with single parents for over three decades, we understand the pressures and challenges of their life. A single parent faces double duty with the care and responsibility of nurturing a baby, while often wearing several hats as homemaker and provider.

Yet, we also know that if you are a single parent, you will love your baby with the same passion as any couple, and will desire to give your baby the best chance in life. It is our joy to help all parents maximize their emotional and intellectual resources, regardless of their marital status. If you are a single parent, please know that while you may feel out of place in various group settings, when it comes to caring for your children, you are always welcome in our community.

SUMMARY

In parenting, everything is connected: the beginning with the end and everything in between. That means parents never act in any given moment without their actions having some impact on the future. That is true not just in the role of a mom or dad, but also as a wife or husband. As we will demonstrate in our next chapter, parenting decisions have ripple effects that connect our beliefs and assumptions with our actions, and our actions with outcomes.

Keeping your marriage strong has positive consequences. Parent from the strength of your marriage and you will parent well. If you're interested in additional resources to strengthen your marriage, please visit our online resource center at *www.Facebook.com/BabywiseLife*. This is a good place to connect with new and experienced *Babywise* moms.

Chapter Two

Feeding Philosophies

One day, sitting by a peaceful pond, I found myself amused by three children, their tiny feet scampering back and forth as they pursued the perfect skipping stone. Who as a child, has not, at one time or another, tried to skip a stone across the smooth surface of a lake or dropped a pebble in a pool of water, and then watched as perfect concentric circles expanded outward from the center? The weight of the pebble breaking the surface creates energy that causes an expansion of ripples, but the initial source that brought this energy to life was the decision to drop the pebble into the water in the first place.

There is a parenting principle tied to this metaphor: Every decision made and every action taken as a result of our personal beliefs and assumptions, sets in motion rippling effects of corresponding outcomes. Those outcomes are tied to the nature of our beliefs.

Our actions affect not only the seen, but also the unseen, often producing unintended consequences. The stone hitting the water, for example, could scare baby turtles floating near the surface, driving them into deep water, possibly toward a predator; the sound of the splash might startle some water birds and cause them to take flight, leaving behind a familiar habitat that provides food and safety. If these collateral actions take place, they are all connected back to us, because of a single, momentary decision to throw a pebble in the first place.

Ripple Effects of Feeding

You would think that establishing good feeding habits would be the easiest part of infant care, since a newborn's drive to satisfy hunger is one of the strongest in life. On the surface it all sounds fairly simple: Baby is hungry, so you feed him. What more do you need to know? Unfortunately, it is not that clear-cut.

When it comes to babies, the ripple effect principle is clearly evident in something as basic as how and when to feed a baby. As we will demonstrate in this and other chapters, the feeding philosophy a mother and father decide to implement will produce an ever-expanding series of ripples that impact every aspect of a baby's life. Every parenting philosophy has its own pathology and will take parents in different directions and to different outcomes. Every feeding philosophy brings with it a different set of parenting priorities and opinions about what is best for a baby, although there is no consensus about what *best* means or how it is achieved. That is because each parenting priority is driven by larger worldviews and beliefs about children, their origin, nature, and basic needs. Different priorities inevitably lead parents to different strategies of care and, correspondingly, to different outcomes.

Unfortunately, as the goals and priorities of each philosophy, are presented, they all sound noble and persuasive, but the outcomes are not equal. The more parents understand each feeding philosophy, the better prepared they will be to make an informed decision for their baby's benefit. Let's examine the three most prominent feeding philosophies in our society and find out what they can teach us about today's parenting theories.

THE EVOLUTION OF FEEDING PHILOSOPHIES

Prior to the rise of early-childhood theories in the 20th century, common sense guided parents with sound thinking, producing predictable outcomes. Mothers nursed their babies based on hunger cues, but also in sync with Mom's daily household duties. Routine was very much part of her day, and routine feedings were part of her baby's life. Today, there is not only a variety of feeding philosophies for parents to navigate through, but each philosophy has its own lingo.

For example, during pregnancy you may have been encouraged to *demand-feed* your baby or warned not to follow a *schedule*, especially if you intend to breastfeed. Maybe you heard about a *demand schedule* or a *self-regulating schedule*. Perhaps you were encouraged to consider *natural feeding* while avoiding *hyperscheduling*. Of course, *hyperscheduling* is rigid, and *rigid feeding* is not as good as *cry feeding*. But the latter is less desirable than *cue feeding*, which is similar to *responsive feeding*. And last but not least, is *bottle feeding*. Where in the world does this fit in? Let's see if we can make some sense of all these titles by stepping back to the last century and examining the origin of today's feeding philosophies.

Philosophy of Behaviorism: Clock Feeding

While the 19th century witnessed a surge in child development theories, it was not until the 20th century that two competing schools of thought captured the public's attention. The first was the behavioral school, emerging in the early 1900s. Behaviorists emphasized environmental stimuli as the primary influence on human behavior. At the same time they downplayed the influence on internal factors such as emotions, human will and human nature. They believed that if you could control the environmental influences, you could engineer the perfect child.

Behaviorism received an unintentional boost with the growing women's movement of the 1920s, which was symbolized by short hair, short skirts, contraceptives, cigarettes, and bottle feeding replacing breastfeeding. The latter became possible because of the discovery of an algebraic equation called *baby-formula*. Since "formula" could be offered anytime, a new feeding practice emerged called schedule feeding or "clock feeding."

A regimented feeding schedule of every 4 hours was considered to be in the best interest of the child, and every "good" mother was expected to follow it to the minute. The baby who showed signs of hunger sooner than 4 hours was left to "cry it out" because the clock, not the baby, determined when feedings occurred with little regard to the baby's immediate needs or the parents' natural inclination to intervene.(1)

The Philosophy of Neo-primitivism: Child-Led Feeding

By the mid-1940s, a second theory, an adaptation of Sigmund Freud's views, started to nudge the rigidity of behaviorism from center stage. A small group of Freud's 20th century followers put forth the idea that children are born psychologically damaged as a result of the *birthing process*. Working within the void of limited science of the day, it was speculated that labor and delivery was so traumatizing to the unborn child that birthing became the wellspring of all future mental imbalances and insecurities.

Otto Rank was the Austrian psychoanalyst credited as the first champion of the *birth-trauma* view (1929). While his theory did not catch on right away, it eventually inspired the *Neo-primitivistic* school of child development, supported by Ribble (1944), Aldrich (1945), Frank (1945) and Trainham, Pilafian, and Kraft (1945). The title "Neoprimitivistic" is not name-calling, but reflects a specific school of thought that postulates that the separation at birth disrupts the in-utero relational harmony between mother and child. Therefore, the primary goal of early parenting is to *re-establish* or *re-attach* the baby, emotionally speaking.

The theory works from a bizarre two-fold assumption that babies in the womb have a perfect "emotional" relationship with their mothers, but lose emotional attachment during the birthing process. This leads to a second assumption: that every newborn has a lingering, subconscious desire to return to the security of his mother's womb. Since that cannot happen physically, the mother is to create and mimic an artificial womb-like environment, and maintain it long after birth. All of her efforts are aimed at reversing the *psychic shock* brought on by the trauma of birth.

From this theory came very specific re-attachment protocols. The process of re-attaching the baby emotionally requires the day-and-night presence and availability of the mother, who is urged to return to a "primitive style" of nurturing.(2) "The baby should be endlessly cradled, sleep with the mother, be breastfed well into the second or third year. The child is to be the center of the family universe, where all practices minister to his comfort and minimize his anxiety."(3)

By 1949, the birth-trauma theory, lacking objective verifiable data, was dismissed with considerable skepticism. Around the same time, the school of behaviorism, while still strong, was beginning to lose influence, in part due to an up-and-coming pediatrician, whose first book sold 50 million copies in the span of his life. His name was Dr. Benjamin Spock; his book was *Baby and Child Care*. By today's standards, Dr. Spock was a centrist and best known for advocating common-sense parenting, while stressing that babies are individuals better served with a flexible routine then a fixed schedule. He rejected behavioristic one-size-fits-all dictates on everything from strict feeding schedules to potty training, but also dismissed the child-centered extremes of Neo-primitivism, which rejected all aspects of structure and routine.(4)

By the 1980s, however, Dr. Spock's centrist influence began to erode because of social conservatives, who thought his views were too permissive, and social liberals, who declared his parenting advice too controlling. With the polarization of Spock's views and the decline of his popularity, there came a resurgence of the birth-trauma theory.

While the foundational tenants of the 1940s birth-trauma theory did not change, the modern version took on a new name. Today it is referred to as *Attachment Parenting*, which in truth has very little connection to the theories of *infant attachment*. They are linked in name only, not by science. It is important to note the distinctions here. The theory of infant attachment is the accepted belief that physical touch is a significant necessity of survival.

As authors, we believe that human touch is a baby's first language, communicating love and security through the portal of the senses. "Touch" is as important as proper nutrition, and the lack of either will lead to failure to thrive.

Parents should minister to the actual needs and vulnerabilities of their babies; however, they should be cautious of any parenting theory that creates extreme or false vulnerabilities. That is when healthy protection turns to unhealthy overprotection to the long-term detriment of the child. Attachment Parenting advocates of the 1980s may have hijacked the name, but they substituted an old, discarded theory for the actual science behind true infant-parent attachment.

Regardless of what it is called today, *Attachment Parenting* or *Re-Attachment Parenting*, it is still the same philosophy, drawn from the same birth trauma beliefs and assumptions originally offered by Otto Rank (1929) and expanded on by Dr. Ribble (1944). Just as it was in the past, the modern protocols for Attachment Parenting continue to be very labor intensive, with a strong emphasis on mothers mimicking the womb; first by keeping her baby in her day-and-night presence—the sling by day and co-sleeping with her at night—and second, through constant and continual nursing, which becomes the substitute umbilical cord.[(5)]

This is why adherents of Attachment Parenting elevate nursing beyond the nutritive value of breastmilk. It is also why a mother can never breastfeed too much, too long or too often, but only too little. Even if it is the third feeding in thirty minutes, the Attachment Parenting mom is acting on the fearful assumption that every cry, if not a signal of hunger, is a potential sign of attachment failure. It all becomes a vicious cycle. Sad to say, the recommended Attachment Parenting protocols required to manufacture a "secure attached child" too often produce the opposite: an emotionally-stressed, high-need, insecure baby and one tired mom.

Creating the Bogeyman

After more than 60 years of speculation behind the theory, there has been no conclusive evidence provided, or a convincing body of research offered that supports the birth-trauma premise on which the modern Attachment Parenting philosophy is based. Meanwhile, the science refuting it continues to grow, especially in light of one fact of nature:

There is no life form on earth, simple or complex, human or animal, in which the offspring spontaneously seeks to retreat to the past in search of an old attachment.

Unfortunately, as long as the birthing process is marketed as a "bogeyman" that inflicts trauma on helpless babies, the Attachment Parenting remedy will always have willful adherents. However, is the womb really a paradise to which the newborn seeks to return? In order to justify the extreme tenants of Attachment Parenting, in this modern age of science, proponents continue to present to new and unsuspecting parents, the birthing process, in horrific, distressing language. They assign to the helpless infant feelings of parental abandonment and betrayal that must be overcome if true attachment is to take place.

In the scientific world, this is known as *apophenia,* (attempting to make a connection where no connections exist). A baby, they say, is born fully conscious of a traumatic upheaval brought on during birthing in which he is forcibly thrust from the warmth, protection, and security of the womb, totally exposed to a new world. In this new world he must exert effort to obtain food, draw his own breath and gasp, cough, and struggle to survive.

Really? Does the birthing process actually do all that? How about a more accurate, rational, *life*-giving perspective that acknowledges that it is only *because* of the birthing process that a baby is truly liberated from a condition of incredible restraint? A baby in the womb is unable to express himself or communicate even the most basic needs. He lived in a world of darkness, in a confined sack where the nutrients that supported life began to mix with his body fluids. It was a place where touch was not permitted, nor was there the opportunity to hear the voices of love, care and protection. A baby is saved only by the miracle and beauty of the birthing process that truly delivers him from bondage to freedom, where he can participate in the wide range of human sensations. For the first time he is able to experience the touch of a loving mother and father and to hear the sounds of their voices, as well as the beauty of the songbird. He is able to experience a thousand different rays of color carried on light beams that the womb prevented him from seeing previously. He is free to laugh, move freely, and discover a world previously closed off to him. All this is made possible by the single passageway carried on the wings of the birthing process. If birth is actually a moment to remember, then it is a moment to celebrate—not one to return to restraint and bondage.

Finally, if trauma is attached to the memory of birthing, by what neurologic function is this achieved? Here is a fact to consider:

Newborns have zero memory of birth, let alone the ability to recall anxiety that is specific to a prebirth experience.

Neuronal development and memory function depend on the brain receiving highly-oxygenated blood, which comes from breathing. Breathing cannot begin until the lungs inflate, which occurs after, not during, the birth process. Higher brain centers that control memory are still developing at the time of birth and afterwards. Thus, where do the facts lead?

While Behaviorists emphasize outward structure and not the inner person, the Neo-primitivists emphasize the inner person at the expense of outward structure. We believe both approaches are extreme and detrimental to healthy parenting outcomes. There is a better way; it is found in the center.

THE BABYWISE ALTERNATIVE: PARENT-DIRECTED FEEDING

While some mothers thrive emotionally on attachment-style parenting, that is not the case for most women. A more user-friendly, less-fatiguing methodology is called *Parent-Directed Feeding (PDF)*. *PDF* is an infant-management strategy that helps mothers to connect with their babies and babies to connect with everyone in the family.

PDF is the center point between hyper-scheduling and the re-attachment theories. It has enough structure to bring security and order to a baby's world, yet enough flexibility to give Mom the freedom to respond to any need at any time. It is a proactive style of parenting that helps foster healthy growth and optimal development. For example, a baby cannot maximize learning without experiencing optimal alertness, and he can only experience optimal alertness with optimal sleep. Optimal sleep is tied to good naps and established nighttime sleep. These advanced levels of sleep are the end result of consistent feedings. Consistent feedings come from establishing a healthy routine. *PDF* is the pebble that creates the ripple effect leading to all these outcomes, including true parent-child attachment.

Embedded in the parent-directed strategy is a critical element for all aspects of infant care: *Parental Assessment*, an acquired confidence to think, evaluate and intuitively learn what a baby needs and how to meet specific needs at specific times. What are the advantages of the parent-directed approach? The following comparative analysis of the three common feeding philosophies answers that question and more!

COMPARATIVE ANALYSIS OF FEEDING PHILOSOPHIES

The three prominent feeding philosophies include:

- *Child-Led Feeding* (also known as cue feeding, demand feeding, response feeding, ad lib, and self-regulating feeding)
- *Clock Feeding* (also known as fixed-scheduling)
- *Babywise Parent-Directed Feeding* (*PDF*)

Theories in Practice

Child-Led Feeding: Feeding times are guided strictly by a single *variable*: the presence of a baby's hunger cues (sucking sounds, hands moving toward mouth, slight whimpering or crying). The hunger cue is considered a variable because feeding times are random and unpredictable. For example, 3 hours may pass between feedings, then 1 hour, followed by 20 minutes, then 4 hours. It might also be "clusters of feeding" such as five short nursing periods in 3 hours, followed by a long stretch of no feedings. Either way, the time between feedings is not considered important because the theory insists that parents submit to any cue that looks like hunger, regardless of the lapse of time.

Clock Feeding: Feeding times are guided strictly by the *constant* of time, as measured by the clock. The clock determines when and how often a baby is fed, usually on fixed intervals of time. Looking for hunger cues is not considered important, since feeding times are always predictable. The clock thinks for the parent (and the baby), and the parent's role is to be submissive to the clock.

Parent-Directed Feeding: Both the *variable* of the hunger cue and the *constant* of time are viewed as necessary tools of assessment.

THE CONFLICT BETWEEN THE VARIABLE AND CONSTANT

The greatest tension with feeding philosophies centers on which feeding indicator to use—the variable of the hunger cue or the constant of the clock. The standard Attachment Parenting/La Leche League doctrine insists on child-led feedings exclusively. Therefore, the hunger cue is always dominant. Parents who believe in hyper-scheduling see the fixed segments of time as the final determinant of feeding. Thus, the clock is dominant. The weakness in the logic of these two views becomes obvious when placed into their respective equations. The *child-led* equation looks like this:

Hunger Cue + Nothing = Feeding Time

"Plus Nothing" in this equation means the presence of a hunger cue is the only consideration that determines when the baby is fed. While this seems to initially make sense, there are some concerns related to this particular approach.

Weakness in practice:

1. Child-Led Feeding is based on the faulty assumption that hunger cues, including crying are always reliable. They are not, and that is the primary reason this approach is dangerous. Being guided by the hunger cue only works if a hunger cue, such as crying, is present. Weak, sickly, sluggish, or sleepy babies may not signal for food for 4, 5 or 6 hours and thus, this type of feeding puts the baby at risk of not receiving proper nourishment.

2. Exclusive cue-response feeding can easily lead to infant dehydration, low weight gain, failure to thrive, and frustration for both Baby and Mom.

3. If the hunger cue is consistently less than 2 hours, it leads to maternal fatigue. *Fatigue* is recognized as the Number One reason mothers give up breastfeeding.[6] They are exhausted!

4. The erratic nature of *cluster* feeding throughout the day produces unintended consequences, including excessive fussiness, erratic nap behavior and instability in sleep/wake cycles, all contributing to infant sleep deprivation. The *Clock Feeding* equation looks like this:

Clock + Nothing = Feeding Time

"Plus Nothing" in this equation, means nothing but the clock determines when a baby is to be fed.

Weakness in practice:

1. Feeding based on fixed times ignores legitimate hunger cues by assuming each previous feeding was successful. It does not take into account growth spurts, which necessitate a day or more of increased feedings. The baby who shows signs of hunger after 2 hours is put off until the next scheduled feeding, and that extra hour usually comes with crying that could have been avoided.

2. Strict schedules may not promote sufficient stimulation for breastmilk production, leading to the second greatest cause for mothers giving up breastfeeding: low milk supply.[7]

With both *Child-Led Feeding* and *Clock Feeding*, a tension exists between the variable and the constant. This tension is both philosophical and physiological. In either case, as parents are trying to serve their underlying parenting philosophy, they become enslaved to a method. To accept either of these feeding indicators as an exclusive guide to feeding is to ensure a stress-filled and, perhaps, unhealthy infant.

BABYWISE-PARENT-DIRECTED FEEDING

PDF eliminates the tension of relying exclusively on the unreliable variable of a hunger cue or the insufficient constant of the clock. With *PDF,* both the variable and the constant are used as companions, backups to each other, not antagonists to be avoided. Consider the *PDF* equation with the inclusion of *Parental Assessment* (*PA*).

Hunger Cue + Clock + PA = Feeding Time

With the parent-directed approach you feed your baby when he is hungry, but the clock provides the protective limits so you are not feeding too often, such as every hour, or too little, such as every 4-5 hours. *PDF* brings into play the critical tool of Parental Assessment, which is the ability to assess a baby's needs and respond accordingly. Parental Assessment frees a mother to use the variable of the hunger cue when necessary and the constant of time when appropriate. Here are some of the benefits of the *PDF* approach:

1. *PDF* guided by Parental Assessment provides tools to recognize and assess two potential problems with infant feeding:

    a. The breastfed child who nurses so often, such as every hour, may not be receiving adequate nutrition. Using parental assessment, parents not only respond to the cue by feeding the baby, but are alerted to a potential problem with the feedings.

    b. When the hunger cue is not present, the clock serves as a guide to ensure that too much or too little time does not elapse between feedings. It is also a protective backup for weak and sickly babies who may not always provide tangible hunger cues.

2. When the hunger cue is present, the clock is submissive to the cue because hunger, not the clock, determines feedings.

When Parental Assessment is part of the equation, parents are protected from moving to the extremes of feeding.

PDF AND INFANT ATTACHMENT

Beyond the assessment tools just presented, the *Babywise* principles also facilitate a robust parent-child attachment. This is achieved by creating an orderly environment that allows the baby's growth and development capacities to be optimized. The process is referred to as *attachment cohesion* and reflects the hierarchical nature of development, where the maturation of one group of factors must first be established before subsequent systems can operate properly. So it is with infant attachment.

The fact that a baby's biological, neurologic and rhythmical needs are merging with his or her natural capacities means nothing is hindering Baby's upward progress toward comprehensive attachment. "Comprehensive" refers to the total spectrum of growth and development. If an infant is out of sync developmentally, he or she cannot be in sync with healthy relational or emotional attachments.

The Measurement of Infant Attachment

"Attachment" is commonly defined by arbitrary "soft" markers that are so broad in scope and futuristic that they have little value when it comes to measuring true infant attachment or exposing attachment deficits. For example, infant attachment is considered achieved, if at some point in the future, a child has healthy self-esteem, good grades or does not do drugs. As wonderful as these achievements may be, they are too "detached" from infancy to have any relevance. When it comes to babies, true parent/child attachment, must be measured by objective markers relevant to an infant's developmental inclinations. Let's work through this natural unfolding sequence.

The process of attachment has a starting point—birth! Contrary to popular attachment theories, the average healthy full-term infant does not enter life burdened with attachment deficits, rather with specific attachment needs. These needs reflect capacities yet to be filled. If the fulfillment of these capacities are not made a parenting priority, or if their importance is minimized, the outcomes are predictable and can be measured by specific attachment anxiety markers. In contrast, the fulfillment of these basic developmental needs, provide objective markers confirming true attachment is being achieved.

The healthy markers include babies who 1) synchronize their feed-week-sleep cycles into predictable patterns; 2) can fall asleep without a rocking or nursing props; 3) sleep through the night eight to ten consecutive hours; 4) have a predictable nap routine; 5) have content wake-times and are adapt to self-play; 6) are able to self-soothe; 7) are comfortable with a variety of care-givers (fathers, siblings, grandparents).

Achievement in these seven areas provides the lead indicators confirming Baby is not stressed or anxious, but at peace with his or her biological, neurological and relational environment. This is where Mom and Dad's parenting philosophy comes into play. We know a link exists between the absence of these indicators and subsequent pathology of stress. If the attachment-related capacities are stifled or suppressed beyond the timetable of readiness, then the child is forced to adopt coping behaviors, which signal attachment anxiety.

What to Look For

Attachment anxiety is marked by the nine, twelve, eighteen month, or two-year-old, who is not sleeping through the night, not taking regular naps, or cannot nap by him or herself; is unable to self-soothe, is anxious when left alone, or away from mom's physical presence, or not adapt at self-play for sustained periods, and must be nursed for comfort. The sad fact is (in most cases), these are all parent-induced deficits.

The contrasting good news? Each developmental maker that needs to be achieved in order to realize true attachment, are predictable outcomes for *Babywise* babies and parents.

For more on *Babywise* attachment, visit our resource page at www.Facebook.com/BabywiseLife.

Chapter Three

Babies and Sleep

You are in a coffee shop enjoying a latte, surfing the web on your mobile device, while your baby plays contently with his bright orange teething ring, occasionally glancing up from his car seat. Suddenly you hear a total stranger comment, "Oh my, what a happy baby you have, so content and alert." You smile with a gesture of appreciation, but are not surprised by the kind words; scenes like this are not uncommon to the *PDF* parent. What do comments like these have to do with sleep? Everything!

When your baby begins to sleep through the night, people will invariably say, "You're so lucky," or "You've got an easy baby." Neither statement is true. Your baby will be sleeping through the night because you worked hard to help him achieve the gift of nighttime sleep. You deserve credit for your efforts, but do keep this fact in perspective: training your baby to sleep through the night is not the final goal of parenting, but it does provide a good foundation for everything else that follows.

Sleep, or the lack of this precious commodity, is one of the most significant influences on a healthy life. Sleep is critically important during the first year because the human growth hormone is released during deep sleep. Equally important are the quality and quantity of an infant's sleep, because they affect more than just the baby—they also impact the welfare of everyone in the household, making the difference between being a joyful, alert parent or a fatigued one.

Babywise babies are characterized by contentment, healthy growth, and optimal alertness. These babies truly exude happiness—which after all, is tied back to being well-rested. In fact, healthy, full-term babies are born with the capacity to achieve 7-8 hours of continuous nighttime sleep between seven and ten weeks of age and 10 to 12 hours of sleep by twelve weeks of age. But these achievements require parental guidance and a basic understanding of how a baby's routine impacts healthy outcomes.

CAN IT REALLY HAPPEN?

Why some babies are able to sleep through the night early on and others are not, has long been the subject of debate and study. The theories range from simple to complex and from logical to bizarre. Well-meaning friends may have told the inexperienced first-time mom that every child is different. They go on to say that some babies are born sleepers, and others are not. New mothers hope they luck-out and get a sleeper.

Behavioral clinicians suggest that a child's temperament is the determining influence on sleep. They tell parents that some children have an easier temperament and are more prone to sleep, while other children fight sleep. More extreme are the suggestions that some babies, classified as *high-need*, will wake up more often during the night and *low-need* babies sleep longer on their own. Although each statement contains a grain of truth, the statements themselves are outdated. Rest assured, you can and should expect your baby to acquire the skill of sleeping through the night, but rarely does it happen without parental training. Consider the four core "sleep facts."

Sleep Fact One

Babies do not have the ability to organize their own days and nights into predictable rhythms, but they have the biological need to do so. That is why parents must take the lead and create structure and routine for their babies and for themselves.

An infant's feeding routine benefits Mom as well. She is healthier, more rested, and less stressed. She has time and energy for other important relationships: her husband, parents, family, and friends. If there are siblings in the home, the baby's routine provides time for planned activities with big brother or sister. As life with Baby becomes more predictable, Mom can confidently plan the day's activities, knowing she is meeting her baby's needs. Everyone wins with *PDF*.

To increase the likelihood of continuous nighttime sleep, a parent-guided "feed-wake-sleep" routine is essential. The key to nighttime sleep lies in the order of those three daytime activities. First comes feeding time, followed by waketime, and then naptime. The sequence of these three activities repeats itself throughout the day. The more consistent the routine, the more quickly a baby learns to adapt and organize his feed-wake-sleep rhythms. Established rhythms lead to continuous nighttime sleep.

Sleep Fact Two

The *quality* of each activity is as important as the *order* of each activity. To re-emphasize the principle of the ripple effect, the stone that creates the initial ripple is the quality of each feeding. That means Mom must work to make each feeding a *full feeding*. Babies (and especially newborns) are prone to doze off while feeding, thereby taking only a partial meal. When that happens, especially with breastfed babies, the child is not taking enough to satisfy his nutritional needs.

When Mom consistently works with her baby to take a full feeding, it eventually leads to productive waketimes. A good waketime impacts nap time and a good napper is a better feeder. As the quality of each activity deepens, it facilitates healthy nighttime sleep. In turn, optimal sleep in a 24-four hour cycle impacts optimal alertness, which improves cognitive function that increases brain growth, and encourages a host of other neurologic benefits. Where does it all begin? With the first stone, when baby receives a high-quality feeding.

Sleep Fact Three

From birth onward, infant hunger patterns will either organize into stable and regular periods or become erratic and unpredictable. When infants are fed on the *PDF* plan, their hunger patterns stabilize. There are two reasons for this. First, babies have an innate ability to organize their feeding times into a predictable rhythm and will do so if encouraged by Mom's feeding philosophy. Second, the hunger mechanism (digestion and absorption) responds to routine feedings with a metabolic memory. Routine feedings encourage Baby's hunger metabolism to organize into predictable cycles. Erratic feedings or "clusters of feeding" discourage this.

For example, if a Mom feeds her baby approximately every 3 hours—Let's say 7:00 a.m., 10:00 a.m., 1:00 p.m., 4:00 p.m., 7:00 p.m., and 10:00 p.m.—the baby's hunger cycle begins to synchronize with those times. When that is established, daytime sleep cycles organize, and then nighttime sleep follows. The exact times above are not as important as the predictability they represent. There is nothing magical about those times. Parents can start at 6:00 a.m., if that works better for them. The principle here is *consistency* which leads to *predictability*.

In contrast, erratic feeding periods work against a child's ability to organize good feeding rhythms, which creates confusion within the child's metabolic memory. For example, the Mom who follows a *cry-feeding* philosophy may feed him at 8:00 a.m. and 30 minutes later when her baby cries, she feeds him again. An hour may pass and he feeds, followed by 3 hours before the next feeding, then 20 minutes. The next day, everything is different, including the length of each feeding cycle and the timing of each cycle. When there is no consistency in the amount of time between feedings, and this pattern continues for weeks, it is very difficult for the feed-wake-sleep cycles to stabilize. As a result, these babies have difficulty establishing stable and uninterrupted nighttime sleep, waking as often as every 2 hours on a recurring basis. This pattern may continue for two years or more according to some studies.[1] Not surprisingly, formula-fed babies who are not on a routine usually end up with the same results. Take note of the next fact.

Sleep Fact Four

It is not what goes in the mouth as much as when it goes in. Failure to establish nighttime sleep is not associated with the source of food, i.e. breastmilk or formula. Our sleep study of 520 infants demonstrated that *PDF* breastfed babies will sleep through the night on average at the same rates and in many cases slightly sooner than formula-fed babies. This statistical conclusion means one cannot rightly attribute nighttime sleep to a tummy full of formula. The statistics also demonstrate that neither the composition of breastmilk or formula, nor the speed at which the two are digested, have any bearing on a child's ability to establish healthy nighttime sleep patterns.

WHAT'S THE BIG DEAL ABOUT SLEEP?

When a one or two-year-old is continually waking at night, it often reflects two possibilities: misguided parenting advice or misplaced sleep priorities. Unfortunately, these children are forced to exist on a starvation ration of sleep. It is not healthy for them or their parents! Try to imagine what it would feel like to wake up two or more times every night for an entire week. The destructive impact of sleep deprivation on an adult's central nervous system is well documented. Deficits include diminished motor skills, decreased ability to think, irritability, loss of focusing capacity, emotional instability, and cellular and tissue breakdown. That is just a partial list!

Now imagine a young child who does not sleep continuously for 8 hours in any of the 365 nights a year! Is it not possible that many of the learning disabilities common in children today are rooted in something as basic as a chronic lack of sleep? As the higher brain continues to develop during the first year of life, the absence of continuous nights of sleep is surely detrimental to the learning process.

STATISTICAL NORMS FOR *PDF* BABIES

A child's body develops faster during the first year of life than any other time. While babies need adequate nutrition to help facilitate healthy growth, they also require extended periods of restorative sleep. Why is that important? Because babies grow during times of extended sleep!

The kind of sleep a baby achieves determines the true value of his sleep. Half of Baby's sleep time is spent in quiet sleep (Relaxed Sleep Pattern or RSP) and the other half in active sleep (Active Sleep Pattern or ASP). Researchers tell us these two patterns alternate about every 30 to 45 minutes during sleep. Noticeable differences exist between the two patterns. During the relaxed sleep state, parents see a peaceful baby. The baby's face is relaxed, eyelids closed and still. He has very few body movements and breathing is quiet and regular. It is also during this relaxed or deep sleep that 70-80 percent of the baby's growth hormone is secreted. That means healthy sleep habits and healthy growth are connected.

The active sleep state is more restless. This is often the time with both children and adults when dreams occur. The extent to which babies dream is not fully understood, but during this period, a parent will notice their baby's arms and legs stir, the eyes flutter, and facial muscles move—sucking, frowning, and chewing motions. Breathing is irregular and slightly faster.

NO PROMISES, BUT. . .

While we cannot offer any guarantees, we can provide the following statistics that represent *PDF* norms. The following conclusions were drawn from a sampling of 520 infants (266 boys and 254 girls), of which 380 were exclusively breastfed, 59 were exclusively formula-fed, and 81 were fed a combination of breastmilk and formula. There were 468 babies with no medical conditions and 52 with medical conditions detected at birth or shortly after birth. Included in the medical-conditions profile were 15 premature infants. All parents followed the *PDF* strategy.

For the breastfed babies, routine feedings were defined as feeding every 2½-3 hours for the first eight weeks. For the formula-fed babies, routine feedings were every 3-4 hours. Nighttime sleep was defined as sleeping continuously 7-8 hours through the night. Volunteer subjects were drawn from the United States, Canada, and New Zealand. The study revealed the following:

Category One: Exclusively Breastfed Babies

Of the breastfed girls, 86.9 percent were sleeping through the night between seven to nine weeks, and 97 percent were sleeping through the night by 12 weeks of age. Of the breastfed boys, 76.8 percent were sleeping through the night between seven and nine weeks and 96 percent were sleeping through the night by 12 weeks.

Category Two: Exclusively Formula-fed Babies

Of the formula-fed girls, 82.1 percent were sleeping through the night between seven to nine weeks, and 96.4 percent were sleeping through the night by 12 weeks. Of the formula-fed boys, 78.3 percent were sleeping through the night between seven to nine weeks and 95.7 percent were sleeping through the night by 12 weeks.

Category Three: Medical Conditions

Of the 52 infants with medical conditions (e.g., reflux, colic, premature delivery, viral infections, and unspecified hospitalizations), all slept 8-9 hours through the night between 13 and 16 weeks.

As the statistical percentages demonstrate, parents can guide their baby's sleep/wake rhythms quite early and with a high degree of predictability. In addition, 80 percent of the babies in our survey began sleeping through the night on their own without any further parental guidance apart from routine feedings. It just happened. There were some periods of night crying by the remaining 20 percent of infants. Most of that took place over a three-day period and the crying was between 5-35 minutes in the middle of the night. On average it took three to five days for a nine-week-old baby to break the old patterns of waking during the night and to acquire the skill of sleeping through the night.

HEALTHY SLEEP PATTERNS

"How did you sleep last night?" is a question spouses often ask each other. Yet we never ask, "How well was your waketime today?" Did you know that there are different levels of wakefulness? While sleep ranges from a relaxed sleep to fitful sleep, the awake state ranges from tiredness to optimal alertness. Most important is the fact that optimal sleep is linked to optimal alertness, which directly impacts optimal learning. What role does healthy sleep play in the developmental process? The documented fact is that babies who sleep well at night make for smarter children.

In his book *Healthy Sleep Habits, Happy Child,* Dr. Marc Weissbluth, Director of the Sleep Disorders Center at Children's Memorial Hospital in Chicago, references the work of Dr. Lewis M. Terman. Dr. Terman is best known for the Stanford-Binet Intelligence Test.[(2)] According to Weissbluth, Terman's findings (published in 1925) on factors influencing IQ continue to stand unchallenged to this day. His study looked at 3,000 children. In every age category, children who were found to have superior intelligence had one common link: all of them had experienced healthy and sustained nighttime sleep from early infancy until the day they were tested.

In 1983, Dr. Terman's studies were objectively repeated by Canadian researchers and the same conclusions were reached.

Children with healthy sleep patterns clearly had higher IQs than children who did not sleep well.

Dr. Weissbluth speaks not only on the positive aspects of healthy sleep, but also on the negative aspects of disruptive sleep. He warns parents that "sleep problems not only disrupt a child's nights, they also disrupt his days by making him less mentally alert, more inattentive, unable to concentrate, or easily distracted, and by making him more physically impulsive, hyperactive, or alternatively lazy."(3)

Infants and toddlers who suffer from the lack of healthy naps and continuous nighttime sleep may experience chronic fatigue. Fatigue in babies and young children is a primary cause of fussiness, daytime irritability, crankiness, discontentment, colic-like symptoms, hypertension, poor focusing skills, and poor eating habits. In contrast, children who establish healthy sleep habits are optimally awake and optimally alert to interact with their environment. These children are self-assured and happy, less demanding, and more sociable. They have longer attention spans and, as a result, become faster learners.

SLEEP PROPS

The typical infant has the natural ability to sleep through the night sometime by the end of the second month of life. It is an acquired skill enhanced by routine. Sleep deprivation in infants and toddlers, on the other hand, reflects the absence of that skill being achieved. There are a number of possible reasons for this, but at the top of the list are a variety of sleep props—those objects used to help a baby fall asleep or fall back to sleep if he wakes prematurely.

Since sleep is a natural function of the body, the primary *sleep cue* is sleepiness. Sleep props interfere with the process by becoming the substitute sleep cue instead of sleepiness. Now falling asleep on his own is out of Baby's control because it requires a parent's presence to offer the prop.

Some sleep props, such as a special blanket or a stuffed

animal are harmless, while others can become addictive. Here are a few sleep props to avoid:

Intentionally Nursing Your Baby to Sleep

The scenario is all too familiar: A mother nurses her baby to sleep. Slowly raising herself from the chair, she eases toward the crib. While holding her breath, she gently lowers the precious bundle and allows herself to smile. Then, frozen in time, she anxiously awaits peace to settle over the crib before backing to the door. She wonders what she will experience this time: freedom or failure? Hoping to escape, the mother knows that if her baby fusses, she will feel obliged to begin the process all over again. Is it "poor mother" or "poor baby"? Is nursing appropriate for inducing sleep every time sleep is needed? No!

With the *PDF* plan, babies will establish healthy sleep patterns. When Baby is placed in the crib, he is usually awake. No tiptoeing, breath-holding, or absolute quiet is required. He may cry for a few minutes or talk to himself, but he will fall asleep without intervention from Mom or Dad.

Motion and Vibration Sleep Props

Modern mechanical sleep props rely on specific stimulation to lull a baby to sleep, either when the baby is first showing signs of tiredness or after the baby wakes prematurely. The most common motion sleep prop is the rocking chair. The question here is not whether you should rock or cuddle your baby. We hope that happens often! But are you using rocking or a variety of dancing motions as sleep props?

Other similar props include the vibrating crib mattress and the baby swing. Some parents have tried the unsafe practice of placing their baby on top of a vibrating clothes dryer. Of course, when all else fails, there is also the nightly drive with baby in the car seat. The sound of the motor and the vibrating chassis of the car sends Baby to dreamland, sometimes. These sleep props work to some extent, but only until the dryer runs out of time, the car runs out of gas, or Mom and Dad run out of patience!

In the short and long run, putting Baby to bed while he is drowsy but still awake facilitates longer and stronger sleep cycles than if placed in the crib already asleep.

Sleeping with Your Baby

Using any of the sleep props just noted may not be best way to help a child fall asleep and stay asleep, but none of them place a baby at risk. There is, however, one sleep arrangement that has proven very dangerous: *sleeping in the same bed with an infant.* To the point of becoming faddish, co-sleeping with an infant is on the rise. Maybe you are contemplating the practice for your own family. Some theorists will tell you bed-sharing with an infant is the ultimate bonding, attachment, and nighttime breastfeeding experience. It is also deadly! What facts do we know about co-sleeping with an infant?

Since 1997, the American Academy of Pediatrics (AAP), National Institute of Child Health and Human Development, and the U.S. Consumer Product Safety Commission have put out medical alerts warning parents of the death risk associated with sleeping next to an infant. The seven-year study tracked the deaths of over 500 infants due to parents lying next to their babies in such a way that they were partially or totally covering them. Do not be misled by that number; it is a small fraction of actual parental overlay cases occurring each year in the U.S.

The American Academy of Pediatrics public policy statement reads, "There are no scientific studies demonstrating that bed-sharing reduces SIDS [Sudden Infant Death Syndrome]. Conversely, there are studies suggesting that bed-sharing, under certain conditions, may actually increase the risk of SIDS."(4) Further, in 2005 the AAP Task Force on SIDS labeled shared sleep with infants as a "highly controversial" topic, and called the practice of bed sharing as "hazardous."(5)

This is why co-sleeping with infants may be the ultimate risk decision of our day. Infant deaths related to unsafe sleeping practices have reached "widespread" proportions; and every one of those deaths was preventable. Infant deaths from SIDS are tragic, but deaths from parental overlay as a result of following a dangerous parenting philosophy are both tragic and needless. Safe and sensible sleeping arrangements start with Baby out of Mom and Dad's bed.

Where Should My Baby Sleep?

Where should the crib or bassinet be located? This question should be answered before the baby arrives. Will it be in the parents' or the baby's room? There are advantages and disadvantages to both locations. The advantage to having the baby sleep in the parents' room for the first two to three weeks is limited to convenience for the nighttime feedings. Your newborn will need to feed at least every three hours, so the closeness of the crib is helpful. One downside is with all the unfamiliar sounds and stirring noises babies tend to make. This will keep new parents awake, wondering if all is okay with the baby. A second downside has to do with Baby's ability to achieve continuous nighttime sleep. Sharing a room after four weeks can postpone a baby's ability to sleep through the night upward to four months.

If your baby is placed in his own room, and you are unsure about that arrangement, consider purchasing a monitor, which will alert you to any immediate need your baby might have.

SUMMARY

The best and safest way to help your little one fall asleep and stay asleep is the natural way. You do not need costly gadgets, a new car, or risky parenting theories. Instead of a sleep prop, confidently establish a basic routine to promote restful sleep. Feed your baby, rock and love him, but put him down in his own crib before he falls asleep.

Join us online as we continue the conversation at www.Facebook.com/BabywiseLife. with more medical research, real life stories, and insights from experienced *Babywise* parents.

Chapter Four

Facts on Feeding

Cuddles, kisses and proper nutrition: this is a good way to start life as a baby! Cuddles and kisses are the easy part, but what constitutes proper nutrition and where does it come from? Whether the calories come from breast or bottle (mother's milk or formula), what is of prime importance is the tender affection provided during feeding times. There is however, a difference in the two food sources and understanding those differences will help provide the confidence parents need to make an informed decision about what is best for their baby and family. What do expectant parents need to know?

First, feeding a baby is perhaps the most basic task of infant management. A baby's sucking and rooting reflexes are well developed at birth, and he will satisfy those reflexes by rooting and sucking on anything near his mouth. When it comes to a broad comparison between breastmilk and formula, it is no surprise that mother's milk is the perfect food for babies, providing numerous health benefits.

According to the AAP, research evidence suggests that breastmilk decreases the incidence or severity of diarrhea, lower respiratory infections, bacterial meningitis, and urinary tract infection.(1) The Academy also points out various studies demonstrating that breastmilk may help protect against Sudden Infant Death Syndrome, allergic diseases, Crohn's disease, ulcerative colitis, and other chronic digestive diseases.(2) Breastmilk is easily digested, provides excellent nutrition, contains the right balance of proteins and fats, and also provides additional antibodies for building a baby's immune system. We believe there are health benefits to breast milk that are yet to be discovered.

Unlike formula, which needs to be prepared, stored, warmed and packed for every outing, breastmilk is ready whenever and wherever. As long as the breastmilk remains inside Mom, it never goes bad and has no expiration date. There are also health benefits for Mom. Breastfeeding enhances the return of the uterus to its normal size and shape, and often helps facilitate postpartum weight loss. What new mother is not eager to get back into pre-pregnancy clothes? In addition, recent studies suggest that breastfeeding may benefit Mom by reducing the risk of breast cancer, Type 2 diabetes, and osteoporosis later in life.

Breastfeeding Trends

Despite the numerous benefits of breastfeeding, the most recent data from the Center for Disease Control (January 2020) says that "while 47 percent of new mothers start out breastfeeding exclusively, only 25.6 percent continue after six months, and the numbers by 12 months remained stagnant and low."[(3)] Why do so many mothers choose against the nourishment, convenience and physical closeness of breastfeeding? Perhaps the decision to quit becomes a necessity for distraught and fatigued mothers who are unable to cope with the endless demands created by a lack of routine feedings and predictability in the home.

Mothers following the *PDF* method have a different story to tell. A retrospective sampling was taken of over 240 mothers following the principles of *PDF*. The survey showed that 88 percent of mothers who started with *PDF* breastfed, and 80 percent of those moms breastfed exclusively (no formula supplements). While the national average of mothers breastfeeding dropped to 17 percent at six months, a full 70 percent of *PDF* mothers were exclusively breastfeeding after six months. Add to these statistics the benefits of uninterrupted nighttime sleep, and at once you see the benefits of *PDF*.

HUNGER CUES

Responding promptly to a newborn's hunger cue is central to both cry-feeding and parent-directed feeding, but there is a major difference. The *PDF* approach encourages full feedings about every 2½-3 hours rather than a cluster of small feedings. Working to achieve full feedings is a key to *PDF* success.

"Just listen to your baby's cues" is good advice, if you know what to listen and look for. As a baby is nearing the end of a sleep cycle, he will often make little sucking sounds and may even bring his hand towards his mouth and begin sucking. Then the parents may hear a slight whimpering, which can grow into a full cry. Those are all cues that it is time to eat, but there is no need to wait until the baby is in a full cry before feeding him, especially if the other signs are present. The hunger cue should always trump the time on the clock.

However, there are some unwelcome feeding cues to watch out for. For example, a baby nursing every hour may be a signal that he is not receiving the rich, high-calorie hindmilk or, equally concerning, that Baby is not getting the quality sleep needed. Remember, healthy sleep facilitates healthy nursing, which in turn fosters healthy growth. Fatigued babies do not nurse well and therefore, will want to nurse more often. Mom's chronic fatigue is another unwelcome cue. When she continually wakes in the morning exhausted from multiple middle-of-the-night feeding sessions, her body is telling her that what she is doing is not working and needs to be changed.

MILK PRODUCTION AND FULL FEEDINGS

If breastfeeding is your choice, here are some basic principles of physiology to understand. First, success with breastfeeding is based on demand and supply (not to be confused with the economic concept of supply and demand). This means the supply of milk produced is proportional to the demand placed on the system. Adequate demand produces adequate supply; but how does one define "adequate" and "demand"? The explanation that milk production is directly related to the number of feedings is only partially true. Certainly, a mother who takes Baby to breast eight times a day will produce more milk than the one who offers only two feedings a day, but there are limits. A mother who takes Baby to breast 12, 15, or 20 times a day will not necessarily produce more milk than the mom who nurses 8-10 times a day. The comparison here is not with the number of feedings in a day, but the quality of each nursing period. Babies on a routine may take fewer feedings, but they take in more calories at each feeding than babies who typically demand-feed with no observable routine.[4] The difference here is qualitative feeding (as with a baby on a routine) versus quantitative feeding (meaning more feedings with less quality).

The *PDF* approach provides for sufficient demand, which also facilitates a baby taking full feedings. Whether you breast or bottle feed, a full feeding at each feeding is one of the goals to work toward. Do not panic if it does not happen at each feeding, but this is what you are working toward.

What are key characteristics associated with a full feeding? The more obvious ones include:

- A sufficient amount of time to receive a full feeding: 10-15 minutes per breast or 20-30 minutes for formula-fed babies is the minimum
- Hearing the swallowing of milk
- The baby pulling away from the breast or bottle when satiated
- The baby burping well after feeding
- The baby napping well

In contrast, babies who snack a few minutes here and there do not derive the benefits that come with full feedings. *Snack feeding* or *clusters of snack feedings* work against a baby's ability to organize and synchronize hunger rhythms. There is also a potential health risk. The more a baby snacks, the less nutrition he receives; the less nutrition he receives, the greater the health risk.

The key to efficient milk production for full feedings is the combination of proper breast stimulation with an appropriate amount of time between feedings. Breast stimulation refers to the intensity of a baby's suck, which is driven by the baby's hunger. The strength of this drive is directly related to the time needed for the milk to digest and for absorption to take place. Typically, infants fed on a 2½-3 hour routine have a stable digestive metabolism and demand more milk than babies who periodically snack throughout the day.

Taking Care of Mom

Nothing is more basic to breastfeeding success than taking care of Mom's nutritional needs, beginning with proper hydration. While it is important to eat a balanced diet with plenty of wholesome fruits, vegetables, grains, protein, and calcium-rich foods, Mom must also take in sufficient liquids. She should not wait until she is thirsty to drink because thirst is a late indicator that the body needs liquids. Nursing mothers should drink 6-8 ounces of water at or around each feeding. Liquids can also include juice, mild tea, and broth. (Beverages with significant amounts of caffeine do not count because the caffeine causes the body to excrete the amount of liquid taken in.) Ironically, too much water in a 24-hour period (over 12 eight-ounce glasses a day) can potentially harm your milk supply.

The warning signs that Mom is not drinking enough water include thirst, concentrated urine (deep yellow), and constipation. For your baby's sake and your own health, stay hydrated!

The Let-Down Reflex

When the baby begins to suckle, a message is sent to the mother's pituitary gland for the release of two hormones: *prolactin* and *oxytocin*. Prolactin is necessary for milk production and oxytocin for the release of the milk. As a baby begins to nurse, he first receives the milk stored in the ducts under the areolae. This *foremilk*, as it is called, is diluted and limited in nutritional value. As the baby continues to suck, oxytocin causes the cells around the milk glands to contract, forcing milk into the ducts. The sensation of milk being released is described as "letting down." The milk that is now "let down" is the *hindmilk*. This high-protein, high-fat milk is rich in calories (30-40 per ounce) and exactly what the baby needs to grow.

Breastmilk and Baby's Digestion

A new mother might come across internet blog posts such as this: "Breastmilk is easier to digest than formula so breastfed babies become hungry more quickly, requiring more frequent feedings" and "Because a baby's stomach empties more quickly with breastmilk, breastfed babies cannot sleep through the night." The first statement contains some relevant truth; the second does not.

Does an empty stomach trigger the hunger drive? No. Efficient and effective digestion and absorption of food does. Absorption, which takes place primarily in the small intestine, is the process by which broken-down food molecules pass through the intestinal lining into the bloodstream. As absorption is accomplished, the blood-sugar level drops, sending a signal to the hypothalamus gland that the baby (or anyone) now needs food. It is a drop in blood sugar—not an empty tummy—that signals feeding time. Therefore, comparing breastmilk with formula has little value in this regard, but comparing efficient nursing and full feedings against numerous snack feedings does.

While it is true that breastmilk is digested faster than formula, it does not mean breastfed infants need to feed more often, but it does mean they need to feed efficiently. Nursing that assures a full feeding provides the sustaining nutrition that breastfed babies need. Moms who follow the *PDF* program will help make that happen. If a mother follows the re-attachment model of breastfeeding, she will experience many, many feedings, not all of which will be efficient or satisfying to her baby.

FEEDING AND HYGIENE CONSIDERATIONS

Most germs are transferred by the hands! When it comes to newborn care, keeping your hands clean by washing with soap and water is one of the most important steps of proper hygiene, especially just before feeding your baby. Washing hands with soap and water for a minimum of 20 seconds is the best practice for lifting out and removing germs. We emphasize the use of "soap and water" over hand sanitizer. While very effective, hand sanitizers do not significantly reduce the number of bacteria on the hand, in part because they are not designed to remove dirt like soap and water can.

The commonly-sited claim that hand sanitizers can achieve 99% effectiveness is slightly misleading, since the claim is based on the product's effectiveness to destroy bacteria on non-porous, hard surfaces and not on hands. When soap and water is not available, and you *do* use hand sanitizer, the Center for Disease Control's public website (http://www.cdc.gov) suggests using products that contain at least 60 percent alcohol for maximum hygiene results.

Washing your hands is not just a good practice for Mom and Dad to establish, but it is one to insist on for anyone who will be holding their newborn. With a baby in one's arms, the natural impulse is to touch Baby's face, nose, or chin or hold and examine his little fingers. While touching is part of the human experience, caution dictates hand washing.

PROPER NURSING POSITIONS

Imperative for successful lactation is the correct positioning of a baby on his mother's breast. Proper latching on the breast requires baby's entire body, head, chest, stomach and legs be aligned and facing Mom's breast. If the head is twisted away from his body, then the baby will not be able to nurse efficiently. Try to imagine sitting in a chair and then turning your head sideways while trying to receive a drink from someone standing behind you. Since your mouth is not centered on the cup, trying to drink and swallow is difficult because your esophagus is pinched at the point where your head is turned. That is what it is like when a baby is not aligned properly on his mother's breast. The uncomfortable neck position makes nursing and swallowing difficult and feeding inefficient. A mom will know her baby is positioned correctly if the tip of the baby's nose is brushing slightly against her breast, and his knees are resting on her abdomen.

Once Mom has her baby's body properly aligned, she then takes her nipple and strokes lightly downward on her baby's lower lip until his mouth opens. Why the lower lip? It is connected to the jaw, which instinctively opens to receive food. The upper lip is connected to the upper face and head and stays stationary when the baby eats. All the reflexes needed to suck, chew, and swallow are in the lower mouth, thus the nursing stimulus is found in the lower lip.

With lower lip stimulation, a baby will naturally open his mouth, allowing Mom to center her nipple while bringing the baby close to her breast. When the baby's mouth opens, the nipple is aiming at the roof of the mouth. A wide open mouth takes in the areola along with the nipple. To further assist in achieving successful feeding, there are three interchangeable nursing positions: *cradle, side-lying*, and *football hold*.

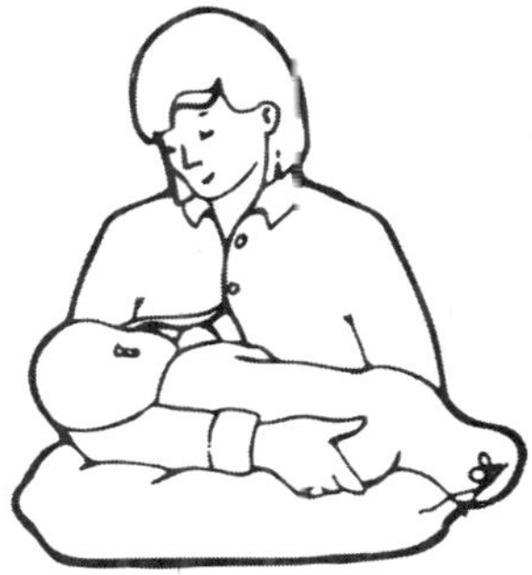

Most commonly used is the *cradle position*. Sitting in a comfortable chair, place your baby's head in the curve of your arm with Mom's forefinger and thumb just below the ears. Placing a pillow under your supporting arm will lessen the stress on your neck and upper back. Remember to keep your baby's entire body properly aligned and facing Mom's breasts.

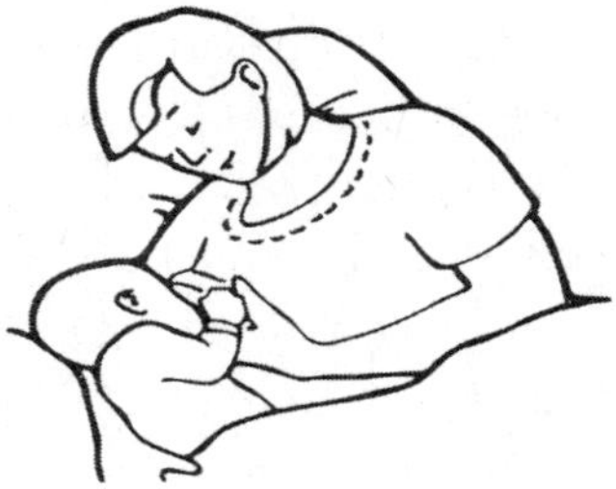

Mothers recovering from a Cesarean birth will often use the *side-lying position* because of their abdominal sensitivity. The illustration shows Mom in a reclining position with her baby supported by a pillow. The baby and Mom's tummies should be facing each other although not touching. The baby's head should be centered on the breast.

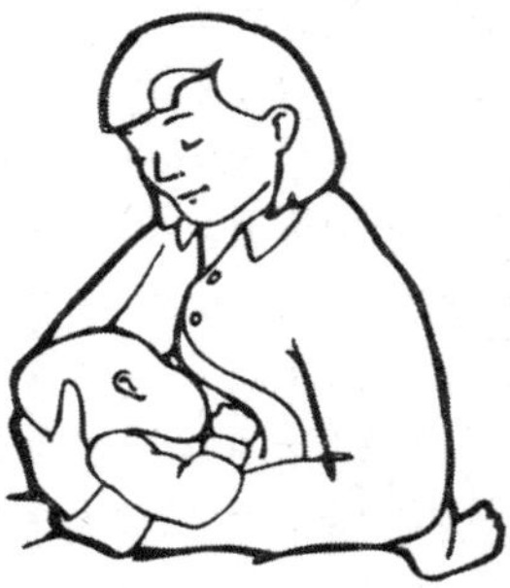

To use the *football hold*, place one hand under Baby's head while lifting and supporting the breast with the other hand. With your fingers above and below the nipple, introduce the baby to the breast by drawing him near. As explained previously, stroke lightly downward on Baby's lower lip until he opens his mouth. When his mouth opens wide, center your nipple and draw him close to you so the tip of his nose is touching your breast.

HOW OFTEN SHOULD I NURSE?

The first general rule is to always feed a hungry baby. How often that occurs depends on the uniqueness of each child. On average (for the first month), babies signal for food every 2½-3 hours. It may be slightly less or slightly more. How do you measure the time between feedings? It is best measured from the beginning of one feeding to the beginning of the next.

There are two components involved—the time it takes for a

feeding, approximately 20-30 minutes, and the total wake and sleep time, which averages 2 hours. Add them together and you come up with your 2½ hour feeding cycle. A 3-hour routine reflects the same components but with a longer wake and sleep time. With these recommended times you will average between 8-10 feedings a day in the early weeks, which falls within the recommendations of the American Academy of Pediatrics.(5)

Can infants adapt or learn to respond to feeding routines in the early weeks of life? Researcher D.P. Marquis compared babies fed on a 3-hour routine, a 4-hour routine, and on demand. The study concluded that while all three groups demonstrated a considerable capacity to adapt to whatever the feeding environment required, the preferred period by all the babies, as demonstrated by their collective outcomes, was 3 hours. Even the babies fed on demand had a natural inclination to organize their feeding times to reflect a 3-hour routine. Babies who were fed every 4 hours, showed a preference toward 3 hours.

One amazing aspect of this study is the year it was conducted: 1941. Here we are, more than 70 years later and the findings have been duplicated, but never repudiated. An infant's natural inclination is to organize his feeding into predictable cycles early in life. One reason the PDF philosophy is so successful is it supports and encourages these natural inclinations of a baby toward routine and predictable feedings.

Time Ranges in a Baby's Day

When discussing time increments for feedings, waketimes and naps, *Babywise* recommendations are given in ranges of time and not as specific times. For example, you will read that feeding times usually fall between 2½-3 hours; and naptimes between 1½-2 hours. It can be tempting to assume the higher number is better than the lower. For example, Mom might assume 2 hours is the better length of time for naps. But that may not always be the case since some babies will tend to nap 2 hours, some 1½ hours and others in between the two. The range of normal times is just that—a range. It is not a scale of good, better, and best with the higher number always representing best. As long as the activity falls within the normal range, it will be the right amount of time for your baby.

While 2½-3 hour feeding cycles provide a healthy average, there will be occasions when a feeding comes sooner, but this should be the exception, not the rule. One of the first breastfeeding challenges is falling into the habit of feeding too often, such as 1½ to 2-hour intervals, or letting the baby go too long, such as more than 3½ hours. Feeding a baby too often can wear a mother down, reducing her physical ability to produce a sufficient quantity and quality of milk. When you add postpartum hormones to that mix, is it any wonder many women simply throw in the towel when it comes to breastfeeding? In contrast, not offering enough feedings during the day because baby's hunger cycles are going longer than 3½ hours fails to provide sufficient stimulation to produce a lasting milk supply. Staying close to the 2½ to 3-hour range in the first few weeks will serve Mom's lactation and Baby's nutritional needs.

THE THREE MILK PHASES

The first milk produced is a thick, yellowish liquid called *colostrum*. Colostrum is at least five times higher in protein, while lower in sugar and fat compared to the more mature breastmilk that has yet to come in. Acting as a protein concentrate, colostrum is rich in antibodies that protect the baby from a wide variety of bacterial and viral illnesses. It also encourages the passage of *meconium stool* which is the first stool the baby passes. The meconium stool is greenish black and sticky in texture, comprising everything collected in-utero, including body hair, mucus, bile, and amniotic fluid.

Within 2-4 days, a breastfeeding mother starts to produce a *transition milk*, which can last from 7-14 days. The content of this milk has less protein than colostrum but an increase in fat, lactose, calories, and water-soluble vitamins. The transition milk is followed by regular breastmilk, known as *mature milk*. The mature milk is made up of *foremilk* and *hindmilk*, which contain different quantities of lactose (milk sugars) and fats. The foremilk is released first from the breast and is generally thin in consistency and lower in fat content, but higher in lactose, satisfying the baby's thirst and liquid needs. Hindmilk is released after several minutes of nursing. It is similar in texture to cream and has high levels of fat that are necessary for weight gain and brain development. There are properties in the hindmilk not found in foremilk that help the baby break down and pass waste, establishing healthy elimination patterns.

A Few More Facts

Once the milk is in, nursing periods will average 15 minutes per side. Breast tenderness in the days before the mature milk comes in is not uncommon. This is because the baby tends to suck hard to receive the colostrum, which is thicker than mature milk. A typical pattern is "suck, suck, suck, swallow." When mature milk becomes available, your baby responds with a rhythmic "suck, swallow, suck, swallow, suck, swallow." At that point, the hard sucking is reduced, and the tenderness should cease.

Another fact to consider is the speed in which a baby will empty the breast. Some babies get right down to business and get the job done quickly, while others take their meal at a more leisurely pace. Studies show that in established lactation, some babies can empty the breasts in 7-10 minutes per side if he or she is sucking vigorously (it is not necessarily gender specific). This astounding truth is not meant to encourage less time at the breast, but is a clear demonstration of a baby's ability for speed and efficiency.

Finally, there are a few factors that can delay a mother's milk from coming in. These include: a c-section, stressful birth, IV-fluids and medication used during labor, premature delivery, maternal diabetes or obesity. In contrast, factors that will influence the establishment of a strong milk supply include breastfeeding:

- Early (soon after birth - preferably in the first 1-2 hours.)
- Frequent (8-12 times per 24 hours.)
- Effective (good latch with effective suckling.)

NURSING CHALLENGES IN THE FIRST TEN DAYS

The length of nursing periods and the span between them will change as the baby's needs change. A healthy start for Mom begins with an appreciation for the miracle of birth and a mother's ability to provide life-giving nutrition.

The Very First Nursing Period

A heavenly drama begins to unfold the first time a baby is brought to his mother and he begins to nurse. It is a treasured moment to be enjoyed, looking into your newborn's eyes, as there will only be one "first" nursing period with this baby. Do not worry about trying to get it right; your baby will know what to do.

Most babies are alert for the first hour and-a-half after birth, making it the ideal time to bring the baby to breast. An initial time of 10-15 minutes per side will allow for sufficient breast stimulation. Remember, the first thing to stay mindful of is the proper positioning of Baby. This not only facilitates proper nursing but helps to prevent soreness. For this first and the next several feedings, nurse as long as you feel comfortable, staying mindful that both breasts need to be stimulated at each feeding.

The Sleepy Baby

After the initial period of postpartum alertness, babies love their sleep. In fact, one of the first challenges new parents can expect is the baby's tendency to be too sleepy to take a feeding. Newborns need to be fed every 2-3 hours, so that means, sleepy or not, Baby must eat! How can you get a sleepy baby to stay awake long enough to take a full feeding? Mom or Dad can remove everything but the baby's diaper and hold him skin-to-skin. Try gently massaging or stroking Baby's face, rubbing his feet, changing his diaper, gently talking or sharing your deepest thoughts out loud. Baby is a good listener and will enjoy the sound of your voice. Be creative and do what it takes to get that feeding in!

Misunderstanding Birth Weight

Although the hours and days surrounding the birth of a baby are usually filled with celebrating and optimism, the first discouraging news comes a day or so later, when parents are told their baby lost some weight since birth. These words strike fear into the heart of a new mother, causing her to think she is not providing her baby adequate nutrition, especially if she is breastfeeding. However, she can take some comfort in the fact that the same thing happens with formula-fed babies.

Although most babies lose five to seven percent of their recorded birth weight (and can lose up to 10 percent and be within the normal weight loss limits), it is unfortunate that this initial drop in weight is described as "weight loss." It makes it sound as if a newborn is actually losing weight that he needs as opposed to losing the extra weight he was born with. The fact is, babies are born with additional fluids and the meconium stool. When these are passed, the adjusted weight reflects the baby's true weight. Dr. Bucknam recommends that parents know their baby's weight at the time of hospital discharge in addition to the birth weight.

Measuring Food Intake

Mothers naturally want to know if their babies are receiving sufficient nutrition to grow on. What should she be looking for? Five to seven wet diapers per day after the first week, three to five or more yellow stools daily for the first month, and consistent weight gain are good indicators that a baby is receiving enough milk for healthy growth. To help track your baby's growth over the first two months, please review the Healthy Baby Growth

Charts in the appendices and fill them in religiously.

The First Seven to Ten Days

Nursing during the first 7-10 days is a time when Mom and Baby really find their equilibrium. These are precious moments and not a time to be overly concerned about the clock, feeding routines, or sleep training. In fact, we encourage parents to turn their clocks against the wall (figuratively speaking), and work on the single goal of providing a full feeding at each feeding. Mothers who work with their babies to receive a full feeding during the first week commonly find their babies naturally transition to a consistent 2½ to 3-hour routine within seven to ten days. The nursing periods for the first couple of weeks may average between 30-40 minutes per feeding. Please note that these figures are based on an average; some newborns nurse faster and more efficiently; others nurse efficiently but slightly slower.

How Long Is a Nursing Period?

Here, mothers have a couple of options. The goal for both options is for the baby to nurse long enough to received the *nutritive* hind milk, which usually averages 15-20 minutes on per side, with burping in between. The second option is to employ a 10-10-5-5 method. Mothers alternate sides, offering each breast for 10 minutes (burping the baby between sides), and then offer each breast for five additional minutes. This second method is helpful if Mom has a sleepy baby, as the disruption prompts the baby to wakefulness and assures that both breasts are stimulated equally.

During these early days, if baby desires to nurse longer, Mom can choose to let him do so. If she feels her baby has a need for non-nutritive sucking, a pacifier can nicely meet this need without compromising the routine or making Mom feel like she is becoming a pacifier. However, we recommend limiting its use for the first month. (You will read more about the benefits and warnings associated with pacifiers in later chapters.)

UNDERSTANDING GROWTH SPURTS

What if your baby is hungry sooner than 2½ hours? Even when Mom has been working to make sure her baby is receiving full feedings, additional feeding times are sometimes necessary. This usually occurs during a *growth spurt*. These spurts are biological responses that affect all babies regardless of how they are fed—by breast or with formula. Actually, the term "growth spurt" is a bit vague and non-descriptive since growth, as it is understood from a length and weight perspective, is not the most visible outcome of a growth spurt.

A growth spurt occurs when a baby requires additional calories for a specific growth need, most likely to restore depleted energy to the body cells that store energy. The extra calories received during this increased feeding times, provide the reserves that support the process of visible growth that follows a growth spurt. Like a car battery that wears down over time and needs a recharge to function at full capacity, it helps to think of growth spurts as the signal that a recharge is necessary. Growth spurts require the baby to be fed as often as hunger cues are present.

For a first-time mom, the first growth spurt can be incredibly worrisome if she is not expecting it, as well as incredibly fatiguing, since it can last any time from one to four days. Fortunately, at the end of the growth spurt, everything returns to normal, including the feed-wake-sleep patterns previously established.

Are growth spurts predictable? There is some disagreement on this. While some clinicians believe growth spurts happen ten days after birth followed by three weeks, six weeks, three months and six months, others say the timing varies from baby to baby. Either way, they tend to fall into a range of time close to what is listed above. Set your cell phone calendar for those weeks with the simple note, "Growth Spurt likely."

For a new mom, the challenge is recognizing the onset of that first growth spurt. Other than a pre-set alarm notice, there is usually no warning before it happens. Just as the feed-wake-sleep routine is finally falling into place, one day she is hit by a growth-spurt snowball! Mom will notice an all-of-a-sudden increase in hunger signs, along with excessive fussiness and waking about 40-50 minutes early from his nap with a ravenous appetite. Mom feeds, puts Baby back down for a nap and the whole thing repeats itself in 2 hours or less.

How will a Mom know when the growth spurt is over? Normal feeding cycles will resume, and the next day, Baby will nap longer than normal. That is because growth spurts are fatiguing for babies as much as they are for mothers.

BREASTMILK OR FORMULA?

When it comes to nutritional value, babies thrive on both formula and breastmilk, but when it comes to the broader benefits, breastmilk is the perfect food. While the nutritional and health benefits differ between breastmilk and formula in the first 12 weeks of a baby's life, the disparity between the two decreases substantially by six months of age. Between six and twelve months, the gap continues to narrow. That is partly because other food sources have now been introduced in the baby's diet. the American Academy of Pediatrics encourages mothers to breastfeed at least a year, which is a common practice for many *PDF* moms.

Breastfeeding beyond a year has value, in that breast milk continues to provide nutrition and immune support. However, if breastmilk is the only source of nutrition at this age, babies tend to become anemic because breastmilk cannot supply all the nutrition that a child needs for healthy growth.

In times past, some tried to make the case that breastfeeding has a higher nurturing value and suggested bottle feeding was an indication that a mother was rejecting her biological role as a woman. It was asserted that her children would suffer emotional deficiencies as a result. Studies over the last 60 years that attempted to correlate the method of infant feeding with later emotional development failed to support any of these claims. A mother's overall attitude toward her baby far outweighs anything else, including the manner of feeding. While the moms who read this book are encouraged to breastfeed, we realize that not all moms can or will choose to do so. One's decision to breast or bottle feed is not a negative or positive judgment on one's motherhood, nor will it have any emotional impact on one's baby.

BOTTLE FEEDING

While formula is a 20th century discovery, bottle feeding has been in existence for thousands of years. Our ancestors made bottles out of wood, porcelain, pewter, glass, copper, leather, and cow horns. Historically, unprocessed animal's milk was the principal nourishment used with bottle feeding. Since it was easily contaminated, infant mortality was very high.

During the first half of the twentieth century, when bottle feeding was in vogue, selections were limited, but today, that is not the case. Store shelves are filled with options, from standard glass and plastic bottles to those with disposable bags, handles and animal shapes. All come in a wide range of colors and prints, although this is more for the mother's amusement than the baby's. The variety of nipples is dizzying, ranging from a nipple that is most like Mom's so the baby feels he is nursing, an orthodontic nipple, a juice nipple, and even one for cereal (which we do *not* recommend). With so many choices, only a brave soul would go to the store without adequate rest or a phone *App* that can explain the differences!

Actually, the only important thing to keep in mind when choosing a nipple is the right-sized hole. A nipple hole that is too large forces Baby to drink too fast, which often leads to excessive spitting up and projectile vomiting. A hole that is too small creates a hungry and discontented baby. To test the nipple, turn the bottle upside down. There should be a slow drip of formula. If the formula flows freely, the hole is too big.

One advantage to bottle feeding is that it allows others to participate. Feeding the baby can be just as special for Dad as it is for Mom. Fathers should not be denied this opportunity to nurture their babies. The same holds true for age-appropriate siblings and grandparents. It is a family affair, and everyone benefits.(6)

Regardless of who is doing the feeding, some of the same basic nursing guidelines apply. Positioning is important. Hold baby with his head elevated. Also, pace the feeding to promote better digestion and allow Baby to take breaks similar to breastfeeding. Finally, do not rush through feeding times, or force Baby to finish the bottle. Similar to breast-fed babies, bottle-fed babies do not always take the same amount of formula at each feeding. That is why a mother or caregiver should calculate the necessary amount of formula required over a 24 hour period, and not just a single feeding.

FORMULA

For some mothers, choosing formula may be the best and sometimes only milk option available. Such a decision should not be viewed as a negative commentary on her motherhood or her parenting. Just as breastfeeding does not make a good mother, bottle feeding does not make a bad one. Moving beyond some other myths; offering formula will not reduce your baby's IQ any more than offering breastmilk can raise it. While breastmilk has many health advantages, formula will not doom a child to frequent infections, obesity or low self-esteem.

The one thing a mom and dad must do when offering a bottle is to take the time to sit and hold their baby. This combines the cuddling that baby needs with the well-deserved rest Mom and sometimes Dad need.

What is Formula?

Infant formula is made to approximate the nutritive qualities of breastmilk. The major types of formula include:

- Milk-based formulas made from cow's milk.
- Soy-based formulas for babies who are lactose (milk sugar) intolerant.
- Hypoallergenic formulas for babies who are allergic to both soy and cow's-milk formulas.

Be aware that cow's milk and baby formula are not the same. Cow's milk is not suitable for children under a year of age. The best source of information about which formula is best for your baby is your pediatrician or family practitioner.

The Food and Drug Administration (FDA) oversees the manufacturing of infant formulas, ensuring the end product complies with nutritional requirements. They are also responsible for recalls that occasionally happen. Baby formula is sold in three different forms:

- Powder: the least expensive form, mixed with water.
- Liquid concentrate: mixed with an equal amount of water. (Easier to work with than powder.)
- Ready-to-feed: expensive but does not require mixing.

How much formula should your baby consume? The AAP provides a handy guide that should be followed. It states babies should receive 2½ ounces of formula for each pound of body weight. For example, if your baby weighs 13 pounds, then he should be receiving approximately 32 ounces of formula in a 24-hour period. Once a baby is sleeping through the night (at least 8 hours), then that would work out to 6-8 ounces every 3-4 hours during the day, but should not exceed the daily portion of 32 ounces, unless otherwise directed by your baby's pediatrician.

Bottle feeding Positions to Avoid

Avoid bottle feeding a baby while he is lying completely flat. (This also applies to moms tempted to nurse in a lying-down position.) Taking liquids while lying down may allow fluid to enter the middle ear, leading to ear infections. Putting a baby to bed with a bottle is also a no-no, not only because of ear infections, but also to prevent tooth decay. When a baby falls asleep with a bottle in his mouth, the sugar in the formula coats the teeth, resulting in tooth decay even on developing baby teeth.

BURPING YOUR BABY

Feeding and burping a baby are inseparably linked because babies will always swallow some air as they feed, and, if the air is not discharged, it will lead to discomfort. Inside Baby's tummy, the swallowed air exists in the form of tiny bubbles that cannot escape or be released without help. Patting a baby's back in conjunction with applying slight pressure to his tummy forces the smaller bubbles to collect, forming one larger bubble that the baby is able to burp up.

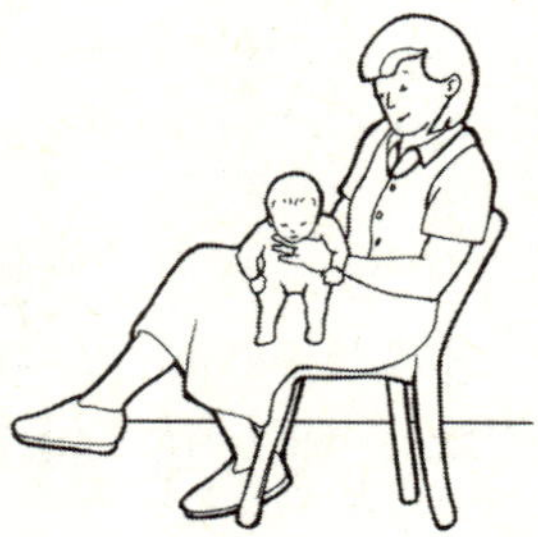

While all babies generally swallow some air as they feed, bottle-fed babies tend to swallow more than breastfed babies. This is because the milk flows faster through the nipple of a bottle, causing babies to gulp air. This problem can be reduced by keeping the nipple filled with milk, leaving no room for air. You may want to experiment with bottles specifically designed to minimize the intake of air during the feeding process. Also, babies (both bottle and breastfed) tend

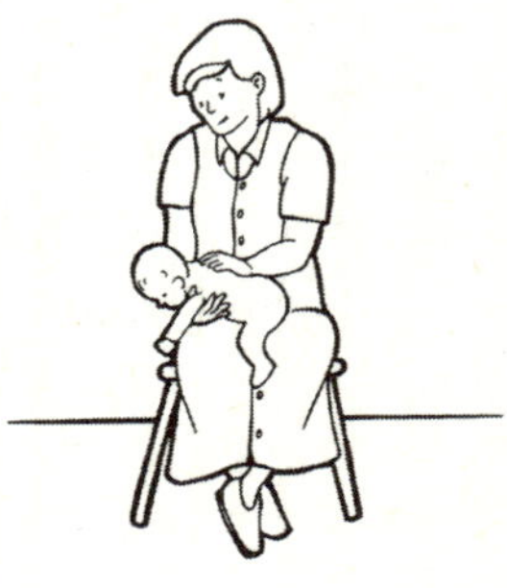

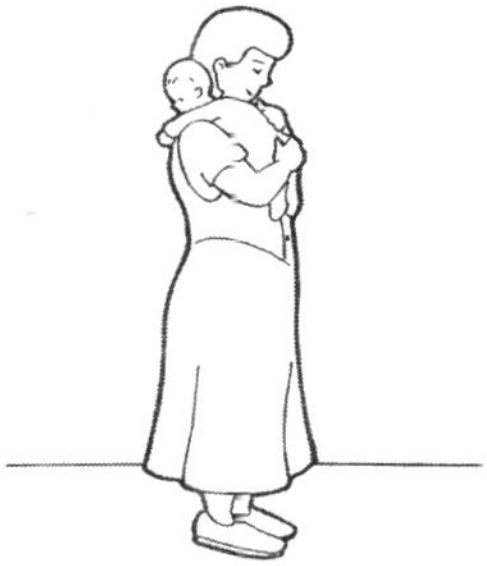

to accumulate less air when fed in an elevated position as opposed to a laying down position.

Burping a baby is one of those acquired skills, so please stay mindful of the intensity of your patting during the burping process. You will learn the difference between a pat that is too gentle or too hard.

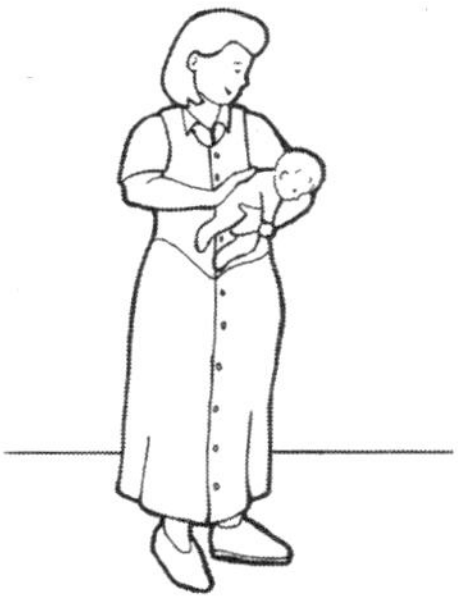

If the pat is too gentle, it will not be sufficient to bring the trapped air up, and if the pat is too hard, it can be injurious and panic the baby. Repeated gentle patting on your baby's back will get the job done—there is no need for excessive force. For more confidence, watch other experienced mothers.

Burping Positions

The four common positions for burping a baby are illustrated, so parents can find the one that is most effective for their baby. What they all have in common is placing slight pressure on Baby's tummy while patting Baby's back. The process of burping may occur one, two, or three times during a feeding, depending on the baby and the efficiency of his feeding. Bottle-fed newborns will need to be burped after every 1-2 ounces, and breastfed babies when changing sides.

1. <u>Sitting Lap Position</u>: Place the palm of your hand over Baby's stomach. Now hook your thumb around the side of your baby, wrapping the rest of your fingers around the chest area. Note how the baby is securely resting upright on Mom's lap with one of her hands supporting and holding his chest. Lean your baby slightly and begin patting Baby's back.

2. Tummy-over-Lap Position: In a sitting position, place your baby's legs between your legs and drape the baby over your thigh. While supporting the baby's head in your hands, bring your knees together for further support and firmly pat Baby's back.

3. The Shoulder Position: With Baby's chest resting on a cloth diaper high on Mom's shoulder and his tummy resting on the front of her shoulder, begin patting Baby's back firmly.

4. The Cradle Position: Mom cradles the baby in her arm with his bottom in her hands and his head resting at Mom's elbow. One of the baby's arms and one leg are to be wrapped around her arm, making sure the baby is facing away from her. This position allows her other hand to be free to pat the baby's back.

If a baby does not burp after a few minutes, Mom should consider changing the baby's burping position and try again before she continues the feeding. Without a doubt, Mom will want to keep her clothing clean, so keeping a birthing cloth handy will have its rewards.

Spitting Up and Projectile Vomiting

Spitting up is a common occurrence and usually occurs during the burping process when the "bubble" is released and some of the ingested milk also comes up with the burp. It can also happen because of unnecessary motion, such as when Grandpa is bouncing Baby on his knee or big sister is trying to soothe Baby by excessive swaying. If spitting up occurs because of motion, it usually signals that a baby has eaten more food than the stomach can process at one time. As the stomach pressure builds, spitting up is the mechanism to release the excess. There is no reason to be alarmed, but Mom should monitor how often this is happening and, if she needs to, reduce the number of ounces her baby is receiving.

A more alarming form of spitting up is called "projectile vomiting," which is much greater in volume and very forceful, traveling 4-6 feet across a room. Projectile vomiting is not a particular diagnosis or condition, but a comparative term to the much less intense dribbling type of spitting up. Although any baby can have a bout or two of projectile vomiting, routine episodes indicate a more serious problem. Projectile vomiting can be a sign of gastroesophageal reflux (see Chapter Eight). It can also indicate an intestinal infection. The baby who routinely vomits his meals will not receive enough calories for adequate growth and can quickly become dehydrated. Establishing a correct diagnosis and treatment is very important.

Burping Challenges

During the first week of life, when a baby tends to be more sleepy, it is sometimes difficult to get a baby to burp. If after trying for 5 minutes, the baby is more interested in sleeping than burping, place her in the infant seat rather than her crib. Gravity is a wonderful thing, helping to keep the milk down and eventually causing the air bubbles to dissipate. After each feeding—with the exceptions of the late-evening feeding and middle-of-the-night feeding—placing the newborn in an infant seat for 10-15 minutes is helpful in preventing the milk from refluxing up into the esophagus. Elevating the head of your newborn's crib by an inch or two can also be helpful, especially if your little one has a mild case of reflux. Simply place a book or board under each leg at the head of the crib.

Hiccups

Even with the best burping techniques, there will be times when an air bubble becomes trapped in a baby's tummy or intestines, resulting in one of two outcomes: hiccups or passing gas. Unfortunately, with the latter sensation, most babies react by tightening their bottoms and resisting the normal expulsion of passing gas, making themselves very uncomfortable. To alleviate your baby's discomfort, place him in a knee-chest position or place his back next to your chest, then pull his knees up to his chest. Every baby goes through a bout or two of hiccups, and some experience them every day, even while in the womb.

Following birth, the sound of little hiccups are actually quite normal (although more troublesome to the parents than the baby.) Hiccups can range from 5-30 minutes in length, and while no scientific certainty can be attributed to the cause, most evidence points to feeding. If you notice your newborn is hiccupping after each feeding, try offering a little less formula or breastmilk, while feeding slightly more often, and see if that makes a difference. Another idea is to treat the hiccups like a burp. Using one of the upright burping positions, gently pat your baby on his back; the release of some remaining trapped air could relieve the problem.

FROM ONE END TO THE OTHER

With new parents, it is amazing how much attention must be given to what is coming back up (burping) and what is coming out (pooping). Be aware that the bowel movements of a breastfed baby will not match those of a formula-fed baby. It is common for breastfed babies in the early days to have a bowel movement after each feeding or at least several times a day. Frequent stools are a signal that everything is working efficiently, and Mom's milk supply is adequate. The stools are usually yellow with the consistency of small-curd cottage cheese. Newborn stools in the first week transition from a brownie-batter stool to a sweet-odor, mustard-yellow color, runny and seedy. The yellow stool is a healthy sign of a totally breastfed baby. After the first week, two to five or more yellow stools along with seven to nine wet diapers daily are signs that your baby is receiving adequate milk for healthy growth. A bottle-fed baby will pass firmer, light brown to golden or clay-colored stools that have a stronger odor than breastmilk stools.

Around one month of age, the stooling pattern for a breastfed baby begins to decrease from several a day to one to two a day. By two months of age, it is not uncommon for an exclusively breastfed baby to go several days without a bowel movement. From our archives of letters, one Mom noted:

> "After my son was first born, I found that he would initially have a bowel movement after each feeding. This pattern gradually changed to having bowel movements several times a day, then once a day, then once every couple of days. Between three and four months of age, he developed a new "normal" of one bowel movement every five days. In contrast, what was normal for our son was not the same "normal" for his siblings. Each child developed his own pattern unique to his own body."

A formula-fed baby tends to have three to five bowel movements a day for the first couple of weeks, decreasing around 1-2 months of age to once a day or every two to three days. The color of the bowel movements can be yellow, brown, or tan, and they are often described as having the consistency of peanut butter. Whether breast or formula-feeding, you will learn what is normal for your baby. The key points are to make sure your baby is passing stools on a regular basis, and to note the color and consistency. For both methods of feeding, the baby's bowel movements should be soft in consistency.

You will find more helpful resources and practical advice relating to feeding and baby-care at *www.Facebook.com/BabywiseLife*. This is a good place to connect with new and experienced *Babywise* moms just like you.

Chapter Five

Managing Your Baby's Day

We previously defined *Parent-Directed Feeding* as a 24-hour infant management strategy designed to help parents connect with the needs of their baby and help baby connect with everyone in the family. The two relevant thoughts contained within this definition include: "24-hour" and "management." The first represents a baby's day and the second speaks to Mom and Dad's involvement in their baby's day—they are to be the *managers*. But what exactly are parents suppose to manage? The short answer is the continually evolving, changing, and growing needs of their baby.

Children come into this world with basic needs for nutrition, sleep, cognitive growth, love and security. As a baby grows, these needs do not change, but how these needs are met will change. Therein lies the challenge. How do you establish a baby's routine that is predictable, yet "flexible" enough to meet a baby's growing and changing feed-wake-sleep needs?

Part of the answer comes from understanding the meaning of *flexibility*. The root word, "flexible," means "the ability to bend or be pliable." To think of a flexible item, think of something with a particular shape that can bend or be pulled and then return to its original shape. Returning to its original shape is perhaps the most critical element of flexibility. During the crucial early weeks of stabilization, it is important that you shape and form your baby's routine. Too much flexibility will not allow this to happen. That is why a baby's routine must first be established *before* flexibility is introduced into Baby's day.

Activities of Your Baby's Routine

The three activities of a baby's routine are *feeding time, waketime, and naptime*. With age-appropriate modifications, these same three activities continue up through a baby's first birthday. The challenge for parents is knowing when the changes are coming and how they should respond. To approach our topic systematically we will:

First: Walk through a year's worth of feed-wake-sleep changes, discussing when they come and how to adjust your baby's routine;

Second: Review specific guidelines associated with the feed-wake-sleep activities for the first 12 weeks;

Third: Introduce some general principles governing routines.

We begin our discussion with the introduction of the *Merge Principle*.

Understanding the Merge Principle

Merge is a very appropriate word in the context of early parenting because the definition describes exactly what should happen throughout Baby's first year. Parental management is all about merging the changing needs of one growth stage with the next. This concept is best explained by an illustration.

On the next page, take note of the sample newborn schedule. There are nine feed-wake-sleep cycles distributed evenly over a 24-hour period. Each cycle, from the beginning of one feeding to the beginning of the next, is approximately 2½ hours in length, which is consistent with the basic nutrition and sleep needs of a newborn. While nine feed-wake-sleep cycles a day sounds fatiguing (and it is), they are also necessary—but only temporary! (The sample times listed on the various schedules found within this chapter, are for illustration use only. For example, we are using 7:00 a.m. as the "first morning feed," but realize your baby may start at 6:00 a.m. or 8:00 a.m. or anytime in between. Personalize the times to fit your baby's needs.)

Sample Schedule
Weeks 1-2

	Activities
1. Early Morning	
7:00 a.m.	1. Feeding, diaper change and hygiene care
_______	2. Waketime: minimal
_______	3. Down for a nap
2. Mid-morning	
9:30 a.m.	1. Feeding, diaper change and hygiene
_______	2. Waketime: minimal
_______	3. Down for a nap
3. Afternoon	
12:00 p.m.	1. Feeding, diaper change and hygiene care
_______	2. Waketime: minimal
_______	3. Down for a nap
4. Mid-afternoon	
2:30 p.m.	1. Feeding, diaper change and hygiene care
_______	2. Waketime: minimal
_______	3. Down for a nap
5. Late Afternoon	
5:00 p.m.	1. Feeding, diaper change and hygiene care
_______	2. Waketime: minimal
_______	3. Down for a nap
6. Early Evening	
8:00 p.m.	1. Feeding, diaper change and hygiene care
_______	2. Waketime: minimal
_______	3. Down for a nap
7. Late Evening	
11:00 p.m.	1. Feeding, diaper change, down for sleep. Allow baby to wake up naturally, but do not let him sleep longer than 4 hours continuously at night for the first four weeks.

8. Middle of the Night
   1:30 a.m. — 1. Feeding, diaper change and right back to crib (Usually between 1:00 and 2:30 a.m.)
9. Pre-morning
   4:00 a.m. — 1. Feeding, diaper change and right back to crib. (Usually between 3:30 and 5:00 a.m.)

Now observe the dramatic differences in the feed-wake-sleep activities of a 10-12 month-old.

Sample Schedule: Weeks 48-52

	Activities
1. Morning	
7:30 a.m.	1. Feeding: Breakfast
_______	2. Waketime activities
	3. Down for nap
2. Mid-day	
11:30 a.m.	1. Feeding: Lunch
_______	2. Waketime activities
	3. Down for nap
3. Late Afternoon	
3:30-4:00 p.m.	1. Snack after nap
_______	2. Waketime activity
_______	3. Dinner time with family
_______	4. Early evening waketime
4. Bedtime	
8:00 p.m.	1. Down for the night

For anyone comparing the two sample schedules, the differences should be obvious. Most notably, the nine feed-wake-sleep cycles for a newborn found in the first schedule were reduced by Baby's first birthday to three major feed-wake-sleep cycles, (breakfast, lunch and dinner). What happened to the other six cycles? One by one they *merged* as the baby developed. The nine cycles transitioned to eight; eight eventually became seven; seven cycles became six, and so on, until Baby's routine was comprised of just breakfast, lunch, and dinner.

The three most urgent questions *Babywise* moms and dads are eager to have answered include:

1. What changes can parents expect?
2. When can parents expect them (on average)?
3. What adjustments will parents have to make?

Every baby is different when it comes to the timing of these merge transitions. We know the average times when cycles begin to merge, but we cannot pinpoint the exact times when they will take place with *your* baby (although the early weeks and months are more predictable than the later months).

Of equal importance is the number of merges. While nine cycles is the average number for most *PDF* newborns, some mothers might feel more comfortable starting with ten feed-wake-sleep cycles. There are some babies who, right after birth, adapt to eight cycles. Regardless of what works best for an individual family, the principle of *merging* is still applicable. Fortunately, there are some general guidelines that can help any parent navigate the various feed-wake-sleep merges.

Guiding Principles to Merging Feed-Wake-Sleep Cycles

<u>One</u>: Understanding the principle of *capacity* and *ability*: A mother cannot arbitrarily decide to drop a feeding or adjust a naptime, unless the baby has the physical capacity and ability to make the adjustment. For example, a two-week-old baby has neither the capacity to go 8 hours without food nor the ability to sleep through the night; thus, at this point in time, a mother should not be thinking about dropping the night feeding.

<u>Two</u>: Understanding the principle of *time variation.* While the length of each feed-wake-sleep cycle during the early weeks of life remains fairly consistent, eventually each cycle will take on its own unique features. For example, for a baby at four months of age, one feed-wake-sleep cycle might be as short

as 2½ hours, while another might stretch to 3 ½ hours. At six months, everything changes again. The range variation depends on your baby's age, unique needs, and the time of day.

Three: Understanding the *first-last feeding* principle. No matter what "merge" is taking place, when adjusting a baby's routine, the first feeding of the day is always strategic. Without a consistent time set for the first morning feeding, a baby may feed every 3 hours, but each day's routine will be different. That is not good for baby or Mom. While there can be some flexibility to this first feeding time, try to keep it within a 20-minute time frame. Remember, flexibility comes after a routine is established. Mom will come to appreciate the consistency of time because she can plan her day around her baby's feeding and naptime needs.

After your baby is sleeping through the night 8 hours, the *first* and *last* feeding of the day become the two key strategic feedings. It does not matter if your baby is on a 3, 4, or 4½ hour routine, *all other feed-wake-sleep cycles will fall within those two "fixed" feeding times and thus, they need to remain fairly consistent.*

Four: Understanding the principle of *individuality among children.* All babies will experience the same merges, but they do not experience them at the same time. For example, Cory began sleeping 8 hours through the night at six weeks of age. Across town, his cousin Anna began sleeping 8 hours through the night at ten weeks. That is a four-week difference. However, by twelve weeks Anna began sleeping 12 hours a night, whereas Cory never slept more than 10 hours a night his entire first year. These two babies experienced the same two merges (dropping the middle-of-the-night and late-evening feedings), but at different times and according to their individual sleep needs.

Five: Understanding the principle of *two steps forward and one step back.* While some feed-wake-sleep merges happen suddenly and take only a day to become a new pattern, most merges take four to six days before a "new normal" is established. For example, during week six, your baby begins sleeping between 5-6 hours at night. By week seven he is up to 7 hours, then, for a few nights, falls back to 5 hours. Eventually he stretches his nighttime sleep to 8 consistent hours and then 10 or more. Two steps forward and one step back is common during the various merges.

Six: The principles work equally well for both bottle and breast-fed babies.

FROM PRINCIPLE TO PRACTICE

What are the developmental "triggers" signaling it is time to merge two cycles into one? For the *PDF* baby, most triggers are predictable and fall into a chronological range of time. Since there are seven major transitional merges over the course of the first year, there are seven major triggers parents should look for.

(Merge One) Between Weeks Three and Six: Most babies start out with two feedings during the middle of the night. For example, let's say 2:00 a.m. and 5:00 a.m. Sometime between weeks three and six, (most between weeks three and four), *PDF Babies* begin to stretch their middle of the night sleep, from 3 hours to 3½ to 4 hours. Consequently, they begin to merge the 2:00 a.m. and 5:00 a.m. feedings into a single 3:00 a.m. "middle of the night" feed. Graphically Merge One looks like this:

2:00 a.m. feeding ↘

Weeks 3-4 → **Merge to 3:00 a.m. feeding**

5:00 a.m. feeding ↗

This merge reduces nine feed-wake-sleep cycles in a 24-hour period, to eight cycles. At this point in time, most *PDF* babies sleep from 11:00 p.m. to 3:00 a.m. They nurse or take a bottle and then sleep until 6:30-7:00 a.m. Sleeping 4-hour stretches at night becomes baby's "new normal." Congratulations, only six more merges to go! (Please note, this merge will be delayed in premature babies proportionate to the number of weeks' gestation.)

Adjustment to Baby's Routine after This Merge: There are no major adjustments needed to the feed-wake-sleep routine during the day. Mom will notice waketimes are beginning to lengthen, but overall, there is no significant change to the feed-wake-sleep cycles. Most babies continue with a 2½ to 3-hour routine.

Sample Schedule After Merge One
Weeks Three-Six

	Activities
1. Early Morning	
7:00 a.m.	1. Feeding, diaper change, and hygiene care
_______	2. Waketime: minimal
_______	3. Down for a nap
2. Mid-morning	
_______ a.m.	1. Feeding, diaper change, and hygiene care
_______	2. Waketime: minimal
_______	3. Down for a nap
3. Afternoon	
_______ p.m.	1. Feeding, diaper change, and hygiene care
_______	2. Waketime: minimal
_______	3. Down for a nap
4. Mid-afternoon	
_______ p.m.	1. Feeding, diaper change, and hygiene care
_______	2. Waketime: minimal
_______	3. Down for a nap
5. Late Afternoon	
_______ p.m.	1. Feeding, diaper change, and hygiene care
_______	2. Waketime: minimal
_______	3. Down for a nap
6. Early Evening	
_______ p.m.	1. Feeding, diaper change, and hygiene care
_______	2. Waketime: minimal
_______	3. Down for a nap

7. Late Evening

______ p.m.	1. Feeding and diaper change, baby back to bed, allowing him to wake up naturally, but do not let him sleep longer than 4 hours continuously at night for the first four weeks.

8. Middle of the Night

______ a.m.	1. Feeding and diaper change, back to crib (Usually between 1:00 and 3:00 a.m.)

<u>(Merge Two) Between Weeks Seven and Ten</u>: Between weeks seven and ten, most *Babywise* babies drop their middle-of-the-night feeding and begin sleeping 8 hours at night. Eight cycles are now reduced to seven. Your baby, however, will not be reducing his daily caloric intake, just rearranging when he takes those calories. He will consume more milk during his daytime feedings, especially at the first morning feeding.

If you are wondering how many hours of nighttime sleep your baby is capable of handling before he needs to be fed again, here is the rule of thumb: By five weeks of age, most babies can extend their nighttime sleep by 1 hour for each week. The average healthy five-week-old can handle a 5-hour stretch at night. A seven-week-old can handle a 7-hour stretch at night.

Adjustment to Baby's Routine after Merge Two: Once Baby merges the "middle of the night" feeding, Mom will need to make some adjustments to the daytime routine. Before Baby was sleeping through the night, Mom fed every 3 hours, which fit perfectly in a 24-hour routine. However, now that baby is sleeping through the night, it appears that the math does not work quite as well with the seven feedings. Here are the new figures to work through: 24 hours *minus* 8 hours of sleep, leaves 16 hours to work in seven feedings during the day. If feedings are divided equally, it would put them at every 2½ hours, so it appears you are moving backward. What Mom wants to do that?

However, there are times when Mom must feed less than 2½ hours. Let's digress for a moment and consider these examples:

- Due to busy schedules, many nursing mothers experience a lower milk supply, quantitatively and qualitatively, during the late afternoon feeding (4:00-6:00 p.m.). As a result, she may need to offer the early-evening feeding within 2 hours of the previous feeding.
- Growth spurts will also necessitate sooner-than-normal feedings.
- When the late evening feeding falls between 8:30 p.m. and midnight, some Moms feed their babies at 8:30 p.m. and then again at 10:30 p.m. The decision to feed within 2 hours is a practical one—it allows Mom to go to bed earlier but does not disturb her baby's nighttime sleep.

Now, let's get back to the time challenges associated with Merge Two. Mom has 16 hours to work with, and she has seven feedings to get in. Here is what we suggest:

First: *Decide the time for the first morning feeding.* Do you keep the original morning feeding time to start the day or do you establish a new one? No problem either way, but a decision has to be made. If you start the morning feed later than what was normal, you could be pushing the late-evening feeding to midnight. Do you really want to do that?

Second: Regardless of what you decide, *schedule seven feedings,* from the first morning feeding to the late evening feeding.

Third: *Remember the first-last principle* noted previously. When reworking Baby's routine, Mom must fit the other five feed-wake-sleep cycles between the first morning feeding and the late evening feeding. However, those five cycles do not all have to be of equal length (and probably will not be); some will be longer and some shorter. Every mom must determine what works best for her baby and herself.

Here is a sample schedule after Merge Two takes place.

Sample Schedule After Merge Two
(Weeks 7-10)

	Activities
1. Early Morning	
6:30-7:00 a.m.	1. Feeding, diaper change, and hygiene care
_______	2. Waketime
_______	3. Down for a nap
2. Mid-morning	
9:30 a.m.	1. Feeding, diaper change, and hygiene care
_______	2. Waketime
_______	3. Down for a nap
3. Noontime	
12:30 p.m.	1. Feeding, diaper change, and hygiene care
_______	2. Waketime
_______	3. Down for a nap
4. Mid-afternoon	
3:30 p.m.	1. Feeding, diaper change, and hygiene care
_______	2. Waketime
_______	3. Down for a nap
5. Late Afternoon	
5:30-6:00 p.m.	1. Feeding, diaper change, and hygiene care
_______	2. Waketime
_______	3. Down for a nap
6. Early Evening	
8:00-8:30 p.m.	1. Feeding, diaper change, and hygiene care
_______	2. Down for a nap
7. Late Evening	
10:30-11:00 p.m.	1. Feeding and diaper change, down for the night.

<u>(Merge Three) Between Weeks 10 and 15</u>: This is when most *Babywise* babies are capable of dropping their late-evening feeding and begin sleeping 10-12 hours at night. (The spread 10-12 hours reflects a baby's unique sleep needs.) When that happens, seven cycles are reduced to six. The morning feeding will remain the same, unless Mom wishes to change it for her convenience, or for the overall benefit of the family. The last

feeding of the night will be fairly predictable because it falls 10-12 hours before the morning feeding.

The breastfeeding mom however, must stay mindful of her milk production. Allowing a baby to sleep longer than 10 hours at night may not provide enough stimulation in a 24-hour period to maintain an adequate supply. While this may not hold true for all mothers, it will have an impact on some, especially those in their mid-30's or older. Therefore, if you are breastfeeding, we recommend that you maintain the feeding that comes around 10:00 or 11:00 p.m. Some moms will continue this feeding for the next four to five months.

Adjustment to Baby's Routine After This Merge Three: Assuming Baby is sleeping 11 hours at night with the first feeding of the day at 7:00 a.m. and the last feeding near 8:00 p.m., Mom must schedule in four additional feedings during the day. Baby's waketimes are significantly longer, although the length of naps may not increase from the last phase, since Baby is receiving a substantial amount of sleep at night. This new phase continues until Baby starts solid foods, sometime between four and-a-half and six months of age.

Sample Schedule After Merge Three (Weeks 10-15)

	Activities
1. Early Morning	
6:30-7:00 a.m.	1. Feeding
_______	2. Waketime
_______	3. Down for a nap
2. Mid-morning	
9:30 a.m.	1. Feeding
_______	2. Waketime
_______	3. Down for a nap
3. Noontime	
12:30 p.m.	1. Feeding
_______	2. Waketime
_______	3. Down for a nap

4. Mid-afternoon

3:30 p.m.	1. Feeding
_______	2. Waketime
_______	3. Down for a nap

5. Late Afternoon

5:30-6:00 p.m.	1. Feeding
_______	2. Waketime
_______	3. Down for a nap

6. Evening

8:30-9:00 p.m.	1. Feeding and down for the night.

(Merge Four) Between Weeks 16 and 24: This is when many *Babywise* babies begin to extend their morning waketime by merging the early morning feeding and the mid-morning feeding. This merge reduces six feed-wake-sleep cycles to five. As a result, there will be only one feed-wake-sleep cycle between breakfast and lunch (although lunchtime is usually moved up at least a half-hour). This is also close to the time when solid foods might become necessary and can potentially impact the timing of activities within the feed-wake-sleep cycles. (A full explanation of how the introduction of solid foods can impact the feed-wake-sleep cycles and nighttime sleep is in *Babywise II*.)

Sample Schedule After Merge Four
(Weeks 16-24)
Activities

1. Early Morning

7:00 a.m.	1. Feeding
_______	2. Waketime
_______	3. Down for a nap

2. Late Morning

_______	1. Feeding
_______	2. Waketime
_______	3. Down for a nap

3. Early Afternoon

_______	1. Feeding
_______	2. Waketime
_______	3. Down for a nap

4. Late Afternoon

_______	1. Feeding, diaper change and hygiene care
_______	2. Waketime*

5. Early Evening

_______	1. Early Evening Waketime
8:00-8:30 p.m.	2. Liquid feeding, down for the night**

* Take note how the late-afternoon waketime activity extends into the early evening, concluding with the bedtime feeding. While there is no full naptime between the two feedings in this feed-wake-sleep cycle, a baby may on occasion doze for 30-40 minutes, depending on when the late afternoon cycle began. This is referred to as a "catnap."

** Possible 10:30 or 11:00 p.m. "dream feed" for the breastfeeding Mom.

<u>Note about "Dream Feeds"</u>: Mothers will commonly ask if there is a difference between the late-evening feed and the dream feed, since they both fall around the same time at night. Yes, there is a difference! The late-evening feeding provides the necessary nutrition baby needs and is part of a baby's routine up through the first three months. The dream feed comes later. It is not offered because the baby needs the calories, but to help the breastfeeding mom maintain her milk supply. Not all mothers need to offer a "dream feed," but the probability increases as Mom's age moves into her mid-30's.

<u>(Merge Five) Between Weeks 24 and 39</u>: Between 5 and 7 months, a partial feed-wake-sleep transition begins to take place, due to the introduction of solid foods and the emergence of the catnap, (a transitional nap, shorter in length, but still necessary). It happens when a baby no longer needs the additional sleep of another full afternoon nap, but is not quite ready to go without a short rest between his mid-afternoon nap and bedtime. Catnaps can range between 30 minutes and an hour, and happen in the late afternoon, usually around dinnertime. Going from a full nap to a catnap does not eliminate a feed-wake-sleep cycle, but moves Baby's routine in that direction.

PDF babies typically drop their third naps and move to a catnap between 24-39 weeks. This large span of time represents a huge variation among babies, yet is a normal range of predictable behavior. It is just a unique fact of individuality that some babies drop the full nap and replace it with a catnap early on, while other babies continue with three naps a day well into the seventh month. Once your baby drops his third full nap, his daytime feed-wake-sleep cycles can range between 3½ to 4½-hours each day. That will depend on your baby's unique needs and the time of day.

Sample Schedule After Merge Five
(Weeks 24-39 *with Catnap*)

	Activities
1. Early Morning	
7:00 a.m.	1. Feeding
_______	2. Waketime
_______	3. Down for a nap
2. Late Morning	
_______	1. Feeding
_______	2. Waketime
_______	3. Down for a nap
3. Mid-afternoon	
_______	1. Feeding
_______	2. Waketime
_______	3. Down for Catnap*
4. Late Afternoon/Dinnertime	
_______	1. Feeding
_______	2. Waketime
5. Early Evening	
_______	1. Early evening waketime
8:00-8:30 p.m.	2. Liquid Feeding, down for the night

* This is usually around dinnertime, (between 5:00 p.m. - 6:00 p.m.).

<u>(Merge Six) Between Weeks 28 and 40</u>: Sometime within the weeks listed, most *Babywise* babies drop their catnap, reducing the five feed-wake-sleep cycles to four, requiring more daytime

adjustments. The four feed-wake-sleep cycles include breakfast, lunch, dinner and a liquid feeding at bedtime.

Again, please take note of the large span of weeks separating *Merges Five and Six*. We previously mentioned the nighttime sleep trends for Cory and Anna. When it came to dropping the catnap, Cory did it at 31 weeks and moved to *Merge Seven*. Anna however, kept her catnap until 39 weeks. That is when she moved to *Merge Seven*. Here are two babies, responding to their individual sleep needs, but falling within the "normal" range for dropping their catnaps. Here is your sample schedule:

Sample Schedule After Merge Six
(Weeks 28-40, *Without Catnap*)

	Activities
1. Breakfast	
7:00-8:00 a.m.	1. Feeding
_______	2. Waketime
_______	3. Down for a nap
2. Mid-day	
_______	1. Feeding
_______	2. Waketime
_______	3. Down for a nap
3. Late Afternoon	
_______	1. Feeding*
_______	2. Waketime
_______	3. Dinner time with family**
_______	4. Early evening waketime
4. Bedtime	
8:00 p.m.	1. Liquid feeding, down for the night

* Baby will receive his cereal, vegetables, or fruits at this feeding.

** Baby joins family mealtime with light finger foods. (This is more of a snack than a full meal.)

<u>(Merge Seven) Between Weeks 46 and 52</u>: This is when Baby no longer receives a liquid feeding before bedtime. He might receive a cup of formula, breastmilk, or juice, but a bottle of

milk is not necessary. Congratulations! You have come a long way since the early days of the nine feed-wake-sleep cycles. Your new schedule will look something like this:

Sample Schedule After Merge Seven
(Weeks 46-52)

	Activities
1. Breakfast	
7:00 a.m.	1. Feeding
______	2. Waketime
______	3. Down for a nap
2. Midday	
_______	1. Feeding
_______	2. Waketime
_______	3. Down for nap
3. Late Afternoon	
4:00-5:00 p.m.	1. Snack after nap
_______	2. Waketime
_______	3. Dinner time with family
_______	4. Early evening waketime
4. Bedtime	
8:00 p.m.	1. Down for the night

SPECIFIC FEEDING AND WAKETIME GUIDELINES

Although we just surveyed a year's worth of transitions, this next section returns the reader to the first twelve weeks of a baby's life and offers specific reminders related to feedings, waketimes and nap times.

Feeding and the First Twelve Weeks

One: During the first week, stay mindful that newborns are sleepyheads, and sleepy babies are prone to snacking: a little food now, a little food later. A series of snack feedings do not add up to full feedings. Baby needs to eat, and the breastfeeding mom needs the stimulation that comes with full feedings.

Two: For a newborn, the duration of time awake, including

feeding, burping, diaper change, cuddles and kisses, will be approximately 30 minutes. Sleep follows the feeding and that takes up the next 1½ to 2-hours. When adding it all together, the entire feed-wake-sleep cycle averages 2½-hours until the cycle repeats itself.

Three: Around the third week postpartum, your baby will begin to extend his waketime after each feeding. This time will eventually extend to thirty minutes beyond feeding. On average, waketime is followed by a 1½ to 2-hour nap.

Four: At six weeks of age, feeding times are still approximately 30 minutes and waketimes begin to increase to 30-50 minutes, followed by a 1½ to 2-hour nap. By twelve weeks, waketimes could be a full 60 minutes or slightly more.

How to Merge or Drop Feedings

Babies "drop feedings" because they are either sleeping longer or staying awake longer. As a reminder, the act of "dropping a feeding" is part of the larger merging process and requires that some adjustments be made in the baby's daily routine. On paper, we can make everything work out, but in reality, babies often need some help. This is where the collective wisdom of experienced mothers comes in handy. Here are a few time-tested suggestions to consider.

1. Dropping the middle-of-the-night feeding: Between weeks seven to ten, most *PDF* babies drop the middle of the night feeding on their own. One night, they simply sleep until morning. Other babies gradually stretch the duration between the late-evening feeding (10:30 p.m to 11:00 p.m.), and the first middle-of-the-night feeding until it becomes the morning feeding.

However, there will be occasions when Mom is on board with the idea of an eight-hour sleep and desires to make the adjustment, but Baby is not a willing partner. He has the capacity and the ability, but sometimes may need a little nudge because his internal sleep-wake "clock" is stuck. You will know this is the case if he is waking within five minutes of the same time each night for three consecutive nights.

There are a few ways to handle this. *One is to allow the baby to resettle himself without Mom or Dad's direct intervention.* Apart from monitoring and periodically checking on the baby, possibly patting him on the back to let him know you are there, allow Baby to learn to resettle himself. Normally, after three to four nights with some crying, the sleep-wake clock adjusts, and Baby begins sleeping through to morning.

A second method is for Mom to push the late-evening feeding closer to 11:00 p.m. or midnight. Once Baby is sleeping through to the first-morning feeding, she can gradually back up the late-evening feeding by 15-30 minute increments until the feeding is where she wants it to be.

A third method, called the *backward slide*, is a last resort. This is how it works: If your baby is consistently waking at 2:00 a.m. each night, preempt this nightly ritual by waking and feeding him 15-30 minutes earlier—around 1:30 a.m. If he sleeps to his normal morning waketime, in a couple of days try moving the time back by half an hour, to 1:00 a.m. You can continue this backward slide until your baby's late-night feeding is at a time you are comfortable with. The way you know you are making progress is if your baby is sleeping from the end of this earlier feeding to the first feeding of the day.

When you are working to establish a new sleep routine for your baby, stick with it. You and your baby will arrive at your goal and you both will be better off when it happens.

2. *Dropping the late-evening feeding:* This occurs around three months and is usually the trickiest feeding to eliminate. Having grown accustomed to sleeping all night, some parents are reluctant to drop the late-evening feeding for fear that the baby will wake in the middle of the night. If your baby is showing a lack

of interest or is difficult to awaken for this feeding, those are good indicators that he's ready to drop it.

The way to drop this feeding is by gradually adjusting the other feeding times. For example, if the late-afternoon feeding is around 6:00 p.m., try feeding the baby again at 9:30 p.m. for a couple of days. Then move the feeding to 9:15 or 9:00 p.m. for the next two or three days. Continue gradually adjusting the time backward until you reach your desired time for the baby to go down for the night. Dropping the late-evening feeding will often make the last two feedings less than 3 hours apart. That should not be a problem providing the last feeding of the day is the priority.

Sleep Guidelines and the First Month

Waking a sleeping baby for food: When should you wake a sleeping newborn and when should you let him sleep? If you need to awaken your baby during the day to prevent him from sleeping longer than the three-hour cycle, do so. Such parental intervention is necessary to help stabilize the baby's digestive metabolism and help him organize his sleep patterns into a predictable routine. The one exception to waking a sleeping baby comes with the late-evening and middle-of-the-night feedings. During the first month a baby may give Mom and Dad a 4-hour stretch at night, but do not let the baby sleep longer than 4 hours. Wake your baby, feed him and put him right back down to sleep. An infant under four weeks of age is too young to go much longer without food.

Waketime and the First Three Months

During the first two weeks of life, your baby will not have a distinct waketime apart from his feeding time. Your baby's feeding time *is* his waketime, because that's all a newborn can handle before sleep overtakes his little body. Usually by weeks two or three, most babies fall into a predictable feed-wake-sleep routine. When this happens, you and your baby have arrived at another level of success. Once you make it through those first couple of weeks filled with new experiences, life begins to settle in as your baby's routine takes shape. What might a feed-wake-sleep routine look like in the first two weeks of your baby's life?

Birth to Two Weeks

Feeding Time / Waketime	**Sleep**
30-50 minutes	*1½ - 2 hours*

2 to 3 hours

Please note the light gray-tone of waketime. It reflects the fact that during the first week, feeding time is basically a baby's waketime. The 30 to 50 minutes noted include feeding, diaper change, burping and any other hygiene care necessary, not to mention cuddles and kisses. Sleep normally follows feeding, and that should take the next 1½ to 2 hours. So the entire feed-wake-sleep cycle will range between 2 and 3 hours, before the cycle starts over. Now note the slight change in weeks three through five.

Three to Five Weeks

Feeding Time Waketime	**Sleep**
30-60 minutes	*1½ - 2 hours*

2½ to 3 hours

Around week three you will begin to notice that waketimes are starting to separate as a distinct activity and may last up to 30 minutes. We are not saying your baby's waketime will be 30 minutes but rather it may last up to 30 minutes in addition to feeding time. Waketime is usually followed by a 1½ to 2-hour nap. With healthy sleep habits established, accompanied by longer waketimes, a new level of alertness begins to emerge that requires additional thought and planning.

Moving to week six, your baby's waketimes become very distinct and the length of feeding time more precise.

Six to Twelve Weeks

Feeding Time	Waketime	Sleep
30 minutes	*30-50 minutes*	*1½ - 2 hours*
	2½ to 3½ hours	

Waketimes are followed by the typical 1½ to 2-hour nap, depending on your baby's sleep needs. By week 12, waketimes could be 60 minutes or longer. By then your baby should be sleeping through the night, so you will be offering one less feeding in a 24-hour period.

However, as waketimes begin to lengthen there is the potential for a subtle and undesired shift in Baby's feed-wake-sleep routine that must be avoided at all cost. Do not allow a "wake-feed-sleep" order to overtake the established "feed-wake-sleep" routine. Here is how this subtle shift occurs. Mom is feeding her seven-week-old, but today, Baby falls asleep without an adequate waketime. After a shorter than normal nap, Baby wakes, but is not interested in feeding because he is not hungry. Trying to keep Baby on schedule, Mom then holds off the feeding twenty to thirty minutes. Instead of feeding after his nap, when he is well rested, Baby is now feeding after a waketime when he has less energy to feed efficiently.

It is not a big deal if this happens once or twice. However, if this subtle shift continues to repeat itself off and on, even for a couple of days, then Baby's routine will begin to reflect a "wake-feed-sleep" cycle. Here is the problem with that routine. Inadequate waketimes lead to insufficient sleep, resulting in shorter naptimes; shorter naps lead to inefficient feedings, and from there everything falls apart. That is why feedings, in the early months, should follow after naps and not waketimes.

SOME GENERAL GUIDELINES: CONSIDERING CONTEXT

Context! Understanding the practical implications of this word will prove to be a valuable tool throughout your parenting.

Looking into the context of the moment allows you to make a decision based on what is best, given the present circumstances. Responding to the context of a situation allows a mother or father to focus on the right response in the short term without compromising long-term objectives. Here are some examples of context and *PDF* flexibility:

1. The two-week-old was sleeping contentedly until his older brother decided to make a social call. Big brother notifies Mom that Baby is awake and crying. It is another 30 minutes before his next scheduled feeding, so what should she do? She can try re-settling the baby by patting him on the back or holding him. Placing him in his bouncy seat is a second option, and a third is to feed him and rework the next feed-wake-sleep cycle. Be sure to instruct the older brother to check with Mom before visiting his sleeping sibling.

2. You are on an airplane, and your infant daughter begins to fuss loudly. The mental conflict begins; she just ate a little over an hour ago. What should you do? The solution is to consider the preciousness of others. Do not allow your baby's routine to override being thoughtful to others. If all attempts to play with and entertain the baby fail, go ahead and feed her, for the context of the situation dictates the suspension of your normal routine. Once you arrive at your destination, make the appropriate adjustments to your baby's schedule. There is your flexibility!

3. You just fed your son before dropping him off at the church nursery and are planning to return within an hour and a half. Should you leave a bottle of breastmilk or formula, just in case? Yes, most definitely! Nursery workers (and babysitters) provide a valuable service to parents. Because their care extends to other children, they should not be obligated to follow your routine to the minute. If your baby fusses, the caretaker should have the

option of offering a bottle. Receiving early feedings a few times a week will not ruin a little one's well-established routine.

4. You have been driving for 4 hours and it is your daughter's normal feeding time, but she is asleep and you only have another 40 minutes to travel. You may choose to pull over and feed your baby, or you may just wait until you arrive at your destination and adjust the next feed-wake-sleep cycle.

Most days will be fairly routine and predictable, but there will be times when flexibility is needed due to unusual or unexpected circumstances. Life will be less tense when parents consider the context of a situation and respond appropriately for the benefit of everyone. Thoughtful parental responses often determine whether a child is a blessing to others or a source of mild irritation.

SUMMARY

How you meet your baby's feed, wake and sleep needs says a world about your overall parenting philosophy. Learning how to establish your baby's routine and knowing when to make adjustments for growth transitions is all part of being "needs-sensitive." At the heart of the *PDF* plan lie three basic infant activities: Baby feeds, baby is awake, and baby sleeps. Matching baby's needs with parental care is all part of the process of learning how to proactively love your baby.

For additional parenting resources, please visit *www.Facebook.com/BabywiseLife*. Connect online and learn how other Babywise moms are managing their baby's routine.

Chapter Six

Waketimes and Naps

As your baby moves from the early days of infancy toward the mid-year mark, subtle growth shifts are continually influencing the various daytime feed-wake-sleep cycles. These small but significant growth changes are difficult to measure in any one moment, but they are present, working behind the scenes, propelling Baby forward. Parents may not visually notice the changes day to day, but they are influencing those changes, especially during Baby's waketimes.

Waketime activities during these early months of life must be understood in terms of a baby's developing mind and his need for proper stimulation of the senses. While waketimes should involve interaction between Mom, Dad and Baby, there should also be times when Baby is alone, totally absorbed in his own world of discovery. Closely tied to waketimes are healthy nap patterns. We will take up naps and nap challenges in the second half of this chapter, but first, before we put the little one down to sleep, let's talk through the various activities that should be part of your baby's waketimes.

MOM OR DAD AND BABY

Feeding: Whether the liquid nourishment is formula or breastmilk, Mom will be holding her baby while she feeds him. Take advantage of these routine opportunities to gaze into his eyes, talk to him and gently stroke his arms, head and face. Touch is important, because it is the first language of newborns and is one they need and crave. Being held communicates security, that their new world is a safe one. While they do not need to be held 24/7 or have constant skin-to-skin contact with Mom, they do need to be held by the many members of their loving community, including Dad, brothers, sisters, Grandma and Grandpa. The more hands that communicate love through touch, the more secure the child.

Singing: A baby will respond to his mom and dad's voices shortly after birth. During waketimes, parents should enjoy talking and singing to their babies, remembering that learning is always taking place. The simple "la la la la la" sound of his parents' voices will have relational meaning to a baby, even though the words do not. Children memorize words more quickly when they can sing them. That means it is never too early to start working with your child to teach him the many different ways words can be used.

Reading: Likewise, it is never too early to read to your baby or to show him colorful picture books (especially cloth, plastic and other durable books that the baby can explore on his own). Your little one will love to hear the sound and inflections of your voice.

Bath Time: This is another pleasant routine for your baby. Mom or Dad can sing, talk and share their most inner thoughts, or just have fun splashing and making the baby's rubber duck quack!

Playing: While smiling, cooing and little giggles are all part of baby play, the best part of a baby's waketime is when he gets to cuddle with Mommy, Daddy, siblings or his grandparents. Such feelings of love and security cannot be replaced.

Walking: The baby cannot walk, but his parents can! Going for a stroller ride and getting some fresh air is great fun for Baby, and walking is great exercise for Mom and Dad. Strollers that have Baby facing outward provide a greater opportunity for learning because he is able to see the world around him. His brain takes in new sights, sounds, colors, and the beauty of nature.

Double-strap, front-pouch baby carriers are another option. They come in a variety of styles, shapes, colors, and fabrics and they are an easy way to take baby on walks, hikes, or when strolling through a store. Look for one that fully supports your baby through his thighs, bottom, and back, and that will distribute his weight evenly to your hips, while being supported by both shoulders. When it is too cold, hot or wet to walk outside, a local indoor shopping mall can be a good place to spend time and explore.

The Infant Side Sling: Since the early 1990s, we have voiced concern about the risks associated with the infant side sling. However, over the years, there have been a number of design improvements that addressed the major risk factors, or at least come with label warnings of the risk factors. Even so, the U.S. Product Safety Commission's original warnings relating to the infant side sling remain to this day.

The Commission notes these two hazards: First, the fabric presses against a baby's nose and mouth, which blocks the baby's breathing and can lead to suffocation. Second, when a young baby with weak neck muscles is cradled in a curved or C-like position, his head will naturally push against his mother's chest. This potentially restricts the infant's ability to breathe and move his head, or cry for help.

Therefore, please read the manufacturer's descriptions and all subsequent reviews. Finally, please keep in mind that there are many safe ways to keep your baby close to you including a variety of safe baby carriers. However, if the infant slings is your first choice, you will find helpful information on the *Babywise.Life* website. All slings listed meet the safety criteria noted above.

BABY PLAYTIME

When young mothers gather to talk and show off their new little ones, it is common to hear differing opinions on many topics, including how best to manage a baby's day. Planning some alone-time into a baby's day is a topic that evokes a variety of opinions. Most parents with an infant in the home tend not to think about this, yet, some monitored alone time provides critical opportunities for learning. By "alone" we do not mean leaving baby out of sight, but rather providing opportunities for him to investigate his world without being constantly entertained. How can a mom make this happen? Experienced *Babywise* Moms will tell you it is a gradual process starting with something as basic as the infant seat.

Infant Seat: This is one piece of practical baby equipment that is especially handy during the first few months of a baby's life. For clarity sake, the term "infant seat" is now equated with an infant car seat. However, we are speaking of a basic infant seat similar to the Fisher-Price® My Little Lamb seat. This style is portable and elevates Baby just enough to view his little world. Parents can find a place for the infant seat just about anywhere. In the early days, the swaddled baby can take a nap in the infant seat. As he becomes more alert, he can join Mom and Dad at mealtimes, or be placed in front of glass door to view the outside world.

The Bouncy Seat: This seat is designed for the baby who can hold his head upright without support, usually at three to four months. It is easy to move wherever Mom or Dad may be. If Mom is in the kitchen, the baby can watch her prepare dinner. If she is folding laundry, the baby is happy to watch this activity and keep her company. The bouncy seat is also great for babies who struggle with a mild form of reflux. Keeping the baby upright 10-15 minutes after each feeding helps her food to settle and minimizes spitting up. Be sure to fasten the safety straps, and never leave your baby unattended. As with all baby equipment, take the time to read the safety instructions.

Tummy Time: Having tummy time on a blanket as part of the baby's routine can begin once he is able to hold his head up consistently, which usually happens between twelve and sixteen weeks. Tummy time is a relatively new concept in newborn care and came into practice as a result of the 1992 SIDS "Back to Sleep" campaign that has babies placed on their backs at sleep times instead of their tummies.

When you do the math on this, you quickly discover that babies today average between 12-16 hours a day on their backs. Compare that to babies a generation ago who slept 12-16 hours on their tummies. As a result, pediatricians and family care practitioners began to notice a significant increase in *plagiocephaly*, which is the medical term for the flattening of the baby's head.

This condition results from Baby spending too much time with the back of the head resting on the mattress. Also observed are delays in the strengthening of the neck and leg muscles necessary for lifting the head, rolling over and crawling, as well as delays in fine motor skills. Tummy time has become a preventive counter-measure to correct the deficiency of the supine sleeping arrangement.

An ideal time to have tummy time is shortly after feeding, while he is alert and happy, but not before a nap, when he is tired and may fall asleep. You can lay him on a blanket or in his playpen. One of Baby's favorite places to have tummy time is on Mom or Dad's chest. Gently move your baby's arms while talking to him and smiling at him. While you are engaging your baby, he is responding by lifting his head and looking at you. Tummy time is a waketime activity you can easily plan into your baby's routine. In fact, it is something you must plan for the welfare of your baby. Most pediatricians recommend 30 cumulative minutes (or longer) of tummy time each day.

Swing: Infant swings have come a long way since we purchased our first one over 40 years ago. Back then they did one thing, swing the baby back and forth. Today, just about every conceivable feature is available, including multiple speeds, various reclining positions and swings that play music as they rock. The reclining option works well if you use the swing after feeding your baby, since this takes pressure off his full tummy. Putting a baby in a swing allows him to watch what is going on around him, but do not get into the habit of letting him fall asleep in a swing. As it relates to fussy babies, they tend to settle better with the rocking motion at a stronger setting and speed. A slower speed is conducive for relaxed, non-fussy times. (There is more discussion related to the infant swing in Chapter Nine.)

Exersaucer:® Once your baby is able to sit up and demonstrates good head and neck control, the Exersaucer is another fun waketime activity to try. This is a contained activity center with a variety of objects to explore, aiding your baby with hand-eye coordination. It also helps strengthen his leg muscles as he pushes and moves in the exersaucer.

The Bumbo Seat:® This is the trademarked name of a product from South Africa (although many U.S. manufacturers have similar seats that are generically referred to as bumbo seats). Its unique shape provides the right support for babies who are starting the transition from lying on their tummy exclusively to sitting up on their own. We find that babies who sit upright tend to have longer sustained waketimes. The longer they are awake, the faster they adapt to life.

Although marketed for ages three to four months, the bumbo seat actually offers no real benefit once a baby is sitting up by himself. In addition, the U.S. Consumer Protection Agency is looking into safety concerns about babies who stretch their backs and slip out of bumbo seats. Common sense, along with the manufacturer's warning, advises parents never to "leave a baby unattended or place the seat in an elevated location such as on a chair or table." It is best to place the bumbo seat on a blanket or carpeted floor, surrounded by pillows and safe play objects in easy reach of your baby.

Playpen: By six weeks, a baby can benefit by spending some waketime in a bouncy seat placed inside the playpen in view of a mobile. As your baby grows and begins to roll over, the playpen will serve as a safe place for waketime activities, especially when Mom or Dad are busy around the home with other children or tasks. The playpen offers a variety of benefits as your baby grows. It provides a secure play environment and doubles as a portable bed. Most important, it is perfect for setting up a structured learning center in the second half of a baby's first year. (You will read more about the playpen in Chapter Nine and extensively in the next book, *Babywise II.)*

Related Waketime Resources

Pictures: All babies are born extremely nearsighted, which means they have difficulty focusing on objects at a distance. That picture hanging on the wall six feet away is quite blurry to your newborn. As each week passes, your baby's eyesight gradually improves and normally becomes 20/20 by the time he is two. You may want to wait three or four months before adding bright colorful pictures to the nursery decor.

Mobiles and Crib Gyms: Moving, musical mobiles help a baby learn to track with his eyes, but first he must be able to focus. Since that takes place about three to four months after birth, hold off until then before introducing a crib mobile. Crib gyms and objects that dangle over a baby and rattle when he bats at them, help to develop his hand-eye coordination. Batting is the necessary preparation for a baby to reach out and hold objects in his hands. For safety's sake, do not place a crib gym or mobile over a baby once he learns to sit up and grab.

NAPTIMES AND BASIC SLEEP NEEDS

Adequate sleep is an important part of a baby's life, and will continue to be beyond his first year. Newborns nap frequently throughout the day, which means a parent can take advantage of naptime for training a baby to sleep when he is supposed to. While parents will not be actively involved in sleep training before four weeks-of-age, they will be doing so passively by establishing a good feed-wake-sleep routine. Below are some nap/waketime summaries highlighting what new parents can expect throughout the first year.

Newborn

Newborns can sleep 17-19 hours per day, which includes the periods of sleep between each feeding. Under *PDF*, this sleep will come in the form of five to six naps (depending on the number of daily feedings). After feeding, when your baby has been up for an appropriate duration of time and begins to shows signs of sleepiness, such as rubbing his eyes, yawning or tugging on his hair, it is time to go back down for a nap.

One to Two Months

By week four, waketime starts to emerge as a distinct activity and by eight weeks it is fully developed. The average nap for the two-month old will be 1½ hours long, with some naps a little longer and some a little shorter. At the end of this period, 75-80 percent of *Babywise* babies drop their nighttime feeding and begin sleeping 7-8 hours continuously through the night. For the remaining 20 percent, continuous nighttime sleep will follow in a couple of weeks.

Three to Five Months

At three months, the length of the baby's naps begins to fluctuate a bit. Most naps fall between 1½ to 2 hours. It is during this phase of growth when Baby may wake early from his nap or suddenly wake early in the morning. The reasons why that may happen and some practical solutions make up the balance of this chapter. By five months, the average *Babywise* baby is taking two 1½ to 2-hour naps and an additional late-afternoon catnap every day.

Six to Eight Months

Between six to eight months, parents will find their baby's daytime sleep needs decreasing as his waketime increases. By this time, the late-evening feeding has been dropped, leaving four to six feeding periods during the day. Nighttime sleep will average 10-12 hours. The baby will have two daytime naps between 1½ to 2 hours in length and possibly a catnap. Once the catnap is dropped, both waketime and often the other remaining naptimes will increase in duration.

Sleep and Nap Summary

What is the right amount of sleep for a baby in a 24-hour period? The answer will depend on your baby's unique sleep needs and developmental age. Nap needs change as babies grow. The chart below is a general sleep guide for the first year. Like most of our guidelines, the averages are based exclusively on the *Babywise* infant population.

Weeks	Time Spent in Sleep	Number of Naps
1 - 2	17-19 hours, including	5-6 naps per day
3 - 5	16-18 hours, including	5-6 naps per day
6 - 7	15-18 hours, including	4-6 naps per day
8 - 12	14-17 hours, including	4-5 naps per day
13 - 15	13-17 hours, including	3-4 naps per day
16 - 24	13-16 hours, including	3-4 naps per day
25 - 38	13-15 hours, including	2-3 naps per day
39 - 52	12-15 hours, including	2 naps per day

NAPS AND CRYING

Naps are one thing, crying is another. The two, unfortunately, will sometimes go hand in hand. While parents should not be anxious about this, neither should they be unconcerned. Here are some facts to consider. Crying for 10, 15, or even 20 minutes will not harm your baby physically or emotionally. Your baby will not lose brain cells, experience a drop in IQ, or have feelings of rejection that will leave him manic-depressive at age 30! That is because a few minutes of crying will not undo all the love and care Mom and Dad have displayed day and night. Who wants a fussy baby who is high-need, never satisfied, unable to soothe himself and living in a state of discontent? That is the inevitable result of "blocking" all crying all the time.

It is a fact of nature that most babies will learn to fall asleep sooner and sleep longer if left to cry for a little while. They will also learn the useful skill of soothing themselves. If a baby is truly tired, his crying should not last long, although if you are the parent listening to it, the cry seems to last forever. Of course, it is hard to hear your baby cry—and even harder to follow through with the decision to allow your baby to cry at the beginning of a nap. Having a right perspective will help, however. Allowing a baby to cry for no reason does not make sense, but when you factor in what is best for the baby, such as healthy sleep training, then crying at naptime has a purpose. It is not a meaningless exercise to test a parent's resolve, but a decision to help your baby achieve the multiple benefits that come with being well rested.

Think of a little crying as an investment toward a lucrative gain. The benefit will be a baby who goes down for a nap without fussing and wakes up rested, and as a result, alert, ready to learn, happy and content. It is a good trade-off for Baby, Mom and Dad. (More on this topic in our next chapter.)

THE FATIGUED BABY

The symptoms of infant fatigue are different from those of a tired baby. A tired baby can usually recoup needed sleep in one good nap or at least within a 24-hour cycle. The fatigued baby, however, has a disruption in sleep cycles that requires special attention. If parents try to keep their baby up and he skips his naps, the problem gets worse. If they attempt to force sleep on the baby by not responding to cries born out of fatigue, Mom and Dad will quickly become emotional wrecks and Baby will still need help. Fatigue is one of those mystery sleep challenges that must be dealt with carefully. Too much is at stake to let this go without proper assessment. Here are some facts to consider when it comes to dealing with infant fatigue.

Healthy sleep has two primary components that most parents are unwilling to give up: a baby who sleeps through his naps without waking and one who sleeps in his crib for those naps. While both are important, one must be temporarily suspended for the greater good of the baby who is showing signs of fatigue.

Infant fatigue is similar to adult fatigue. We all know what it feels like to be so tired that sleep eludes us. Fatigue attacks our sleep rhythms. With babies it prevents them from entering the ebb and flow of active and relaxed sleep cycles. It may come from their routine being out of whack for several days, especially during the time of day when naps are the norm. The priority is for Mom to find a non-stressful solution to reestablishing her baby's circadian rhythm (his normal 24-hour cycle of waking and sleeping).

If you sense your baby needs this kind of adjustment, and you are now in a position to get him back into a predictable routine, we recommend that Mom find a comfortable chair and a good book and allow her baby to take a nap in her arms. This might extend into the next day. On the third day, however, naps return to the crib. This works because the tension between the need and place for sleep is temporarily suspended while Baby gets restorative sleep in the most comfortable way possible. You are not creating a sleep prop because this adjustment is only for a couple of days while you help your baby overcome his fatigue.

Prevention is the best medicine! Try to think through how

your perfect sleeper became a fatigued baby. It did not just happen, and one day's suspension of a baby's routine does not create fatigue, although two to three days of continual disruption probably will. Take a look at what is going on in your home and with Baby's schedule, and make the appropriate adjustments.

THE WAKING-EARLY NAP CHALLENGE

You work diligently for weeks helping your three-month-old establish a great feed-wake-sleep routine; and then suddenly one day, he begins to wake 30-45 minutes into his nap with no signs of settling back down. Why would a good napper do that, and how long will this last? A few hours or a few days? How will this impact the rest of his routine? Is there anything Mom can do to solve her baby's nap challenge?

For expecting parents and parents of newborns, the following section, relating to babies waking early from their nap, is not a challenge they will have to contend with right away. However, this will become a very popular chapter mothers and fathers will return to many times in the future. That is because this section deals with sleep and nap challenges—not the challenge of initially establishing a good sleep routine with your baby, but the challenges associated with sudden disruptions to well-established naptime routines. The challenge is real and there is plenty of help awaiting eager parents seeking solutions just a page away. But first, a story about "Switch 26."

Between 1991-1994 Gary and Anne Marie Ezzo hosted "Parenting on the Line," a live 2-hour radio program. The broadcast studio was fully equipped with satellite feeds, transmitters, relays and a host of dials, switches, and buttons they had no working knowledge of. Fortunately, their radio engineer did. At the start of one broadcast, the normal 60-second countdown began. At the 40-second mark, they realized their microphones were not on and saw the engineer's anxious look as he gazed at their frantic faces. Seconds later, the engineer was standing near them, scanning a bank of 30 tiny switches in various on/off positions. He suddenly fixed his gaze on Switch 26, flipped it to the "On-Air" position, and instantly the microphones were alive.

The Ezzos never forgot that moment or the feeling of anxious bewilderment when their predictable routine was unexpectedly interrupted. Parenting has its share of bewildering moments, such as when a baby wakes early out of a sound nap, contrary to his normal habit of sleep. Like "Switch 26," the fixes are fairly easy, but identifying the cause of the problem is not always as clear-cut, especially if a mother is not sure what to look for.

But what if there was a checklist that parents could work through to help them identify the most likely cause of their baby's nap disturbance? The good news for the *Babywise* mom and dad is that a list like that does exist. On the following pages, you will find a variety of reasons why babies wake early from their naps. At first glance the list might seem a bit overwhelming as you begin to count up the number of possible sources for nap interruptions. Fortunately, the number of possible causes are drastically reduced once parents factor in a few variables, such as Baby's age and primary food source, (breastmilk, formula, and/or solid foods).

Parents will also want to consider the routine nature of the disturbance. Is this a problem at every nap, only morning naps or just afternoon naps? Is Baby waking only at naptime, or is he waking at night also? Does the problem happen every day or once every three days? Basically, you are looking to see if there are any patterns developing.

Of course, this section has little value if the foundations of healthy normative sleep have not been achieved in the first place. We are assuming that Baby is on a well-established 3-4 hour feed-wake-sleep routine, is already sleeping through the night at least 8 hours, and is routinely napping at least 1½-2 hours. These are normal *Babywise* achievements. That is why waking early from a nap runs contrary to what is "normal."

Isolating the Source of the Problem

We have all experienced it. Sitting with our laptop, we discover our internet connection is no longer working. Is the problem connected to our laptop, wireless router, a loose connection in the modem, or a disturbance down line with the internet provider? While the goal is to get the internet back up, we have to discover the origin of the problem.

In a similar manner, nap disturbances can be triggered from a variety of sources. The problem might be baby-related, but it might also be associated with Mom or her diet, waketime activities, or Baby's sleep environment. Isolating the cause of your baby's sleep disturbance is the first step toward fixing the problem. To help with this, our list is divided into four categories. While some causes of sleep problems have obvious solutions (a diaper needs changing, trapped gas or a burp must come out), other causes are more subtle and need investigation.

For clarity sake, we are providing two lists. The first provides a general overview of the many reasons babies wake early from their naps, whether it happens three times a month or three times a day. The second list provides an expanded explanation of causes that impact more than an occasional nap. They are set apart by asterisks (*). Working through both lists can move Mom and Baby closer to the needed solution.

List One

<u>Sleep Challenges Related to Baby</u>

Here are some potential baby-related contributors to Baby waking early:

1. Baby is hungry because:
    a. He did not take a full feeding at his previous feeding
    b. He needs more "milk" calories in a 24-hour period*
    c. He is starting a growth spurt*
    d. He is ready to start solid foods*

2. Baby is uncomfortable because:

a. He is getting sick, has a slight fever, is teething, starting an ear infection, etc.
b. He has an insect bite or a hair twisted around a toe (tourniquet syndrome)*
c. He is too hot or too cold
d. He has a diaper rash

3. Baby's tummy is troubling him because:
   a. He has a mild or delayed case of reflux*
   b. He is having an allergic reaction to a new baby food*
   c. He is struggling with a bowel movement
   d. He needs a burp

4. Baby woke up because:
   a. He startled himself (startle reflex)
   b. He rolled over and does not know how to roll back
   c. He lost his pacifier and cannot resettle without it

5. Baby is starting a sleep/nap transition because:
   a. He is extending his nighttime sleep, affecting daytime naps*
   b. His body does not require as much sleep in a 24-hour period, thus impacting naps.

Sleep Challenges Related to Mom

Here are some potential mother-related contributors to Baby waking early:

1. Baby is hungry because:
   a. The previous feeding proved to be inadequate
   b. Mom's milk supply has gradually decreased*

2. Mom's diet is affecting the nursing baby

3. Baby has a reaction to a new medication Mom is taking*

4. The nursing baby is getting too much *lactose* from Mom*

5. Mom's schedule was rushed, so she did not allow enough time for her baby to receive a full feeding.

Sleep Challenges Related to Activities

Here are some potential waketime activities that can contribute to Baby waking early:

1. Previous waketime was too short*

2. Previous waketime was over-stimulating to baby because:
   a. The waketime was too long, thus promoting fatigue rather than sleepiness
   b. The waketime activity was too over-stimulating (e.g. placing baby in front of TV)*
   c. Baby's overall routine has too much flexibility (e.g., Mom is running too many errands, and Baby is catching catnaps in the car)

3. First feeding of the day has too much flexibility*

4. The three activities of Baby's day are out of order. Mom has baby on *wake-feed-sleep* schedule instead of *feed-wake-sleep* schedule. (See explanation on page 108.)

Sleep Challenges Related to the Environment

Here are some potential environment-related contributors to Baby waking early:

1. Baby is not being exposed to an adequate amount of daylight. Natural light helps babies regulate their circadian clock.*

2. Baby's room is not dark enough.*

3. Baby is over-stimulated in the crib because of wind-up toys

that were turned on when he was put down for his nap.*

4. When your baby reaches four to six months of age, he could be waking up in response to familiar sounds in the home.*

5. Unknown: What does this mean? Simply that a reason exists, but it is so unique to your baby's situation that it is not easily duplicated by other babies.*

List Two

This list contains an explanation of many of the various sleep challenges noted above.

1. Baby is hungry because he needs more milk calories in a 24-hour period.

Explanation/Recommendation: Whether breast or formula feeding, a baby's growth necessitates more calories. While this does not always signal the start of solids, it may signal a need for more feedings (if breastfeeding) or more ounces (if offering formula). Hunger can disrupt established nap and nighttime sleep routines. Check with your baby's pediatrician for literature relating to number of ounces a baby needs at each week or month of life.

2. Baby is starting a growth spurt.

Explanation/Recommendation: Growth spurts will disrupt Baby's naptimes for the length of the spurt, which may be one to four days. When a growth spurt takes place, feed as often as your baby needs but try to maintain the feed-wake-sleep cycles as best you can. The day after the growth spurt ends, your baby will take longer-than-normal naps for a few days. That is because growth spurts are as exhausting for Baby as for Mom. A growth spurt is a biological process in which a baby requires additional calories for a specific growth need, most likely to restore depleted energy to the cells. Your primary concern is to provide the extra calories your baby needs. (Please review the Growth Spurt section in Chapter Four.)

3. Baby is ready to start solid foods.

Explanation/Recommendation: For the baby who has a well-established nighttime sleep pattern, any abnormal waking at night between five and six months of age or waking early during naps might also signal that more nutrition is required during the day. Babies are highly individual when it comes to showing a readiness for solid foods. One baby might show signs at four months, while another shows no signs of readiness until six months. As a general rule, babies usually start between four and six months of age, although some research suggests that holding off solids to five or six months may decrease the possibility of food allergies. Please note, the research is not suggesting that by offering solids at four months you will create food allergies, but rather that some babies have an underdeveloped ability to digest solid foods, which is reflected by food allergies. The AAP leans toward six months before starting solids, but most grandmothers will tell you any time between four and six months is appropriate if your baby shows all the signs. Your baby's pediatrician or family practitioner will direct you based on your child's unique nutritional needs and readiness cues.

4. Baby is uncomfortable because he is getting sick, is teething, has a slight fever, start of an ear infection, etc.

Explanation/Recommendation: It is a little scary! Your baby wakes early from his nap, cries as if in pain, but you do not know why. First, you check his forehead for any indication of a fever. Ears and nose are next. No redness is good news, so you examine the baby's mouth for an emerging new tooth. Nothing there. Examination time is over. You assume it is a sleep issue.

Not so fast! The sudden and unexplainable cry has reason, and as a parent you must figure out why. If you have not already, get into the habit of checking your baby all over once a day, including fingers and toes. Certainly look for the bug bites, which will often show up as a red skin bump. There is also a condition, though relatively under-reported, called "toe-tourniquet" syndrome. A single strand of hair, usually Mom's, or a fiber from a carpet or blanket where the baby was playing, somehow gets wrapped around a toe or finger. Although hardly noticeable, it eventually begins to tighten and cut off circulation to the appendage, causing swelling, inflammation, and pain. The problem is often missed because the baby is wearing a sock or sleeper. While this may not explain every sudden and unexplainable cry or why your baby is waking early from his naps, it does alert you to the need for a daily "once over" of your baby's body.

5. Baby's tummy is troubling him because he has a mild or delayed case of *reflux*.

<u>Explanation/Recommendation</u>: While you can read more about *reflux* in Chapter Eight, it is important to understand that reflux symptoms may not be present at birth and may not show up for several weeks. It is estimated that in the United States, three to five percent of all newborns have mild to severe reflux symptoms for the first few months of life. Reflux is the result of an immature sphincter valve where the esophagus connects with the stomach. When working properly, it opens to allow us to swallow, burp or vomit, then closes immediately afterward. Reflux occurs when the sphincter stays relaxed or relaxes periodically, allowing food mixed with stomach acid to back up into the esophagus and throat, causing pain. This condition is called heartburn in the adult world.

If your baby is troubled by reflux, you can count on it showing up throughout the day, not just at naptime. We have a little friend named Micah, who provides an example of this. After three weeks, a mild case of reflux began to manifest itself. To counter its effects, his parents did two things: They kept him upright for a short time following each feeding, and they elevated the head of his crib by two inches, allowing gravity to prevent stomach acids from moving back into Micah's esophagus while he was sleeping. Because this was a mild case of reflux, these solutions worked. For more severe cases, medication may be necessary.

6. Your baby is having an on-going allergic reaction to a new baby food.

Explanation/Recommendation: One basic rule of introducing solids is to begin with one item at a time, waiting three to five days before introducing another new food type to see if your baby develops an allergic reaction. Sequential introduction of food items allows you to monitor your baby's reaction so proper nutritional adjustments can be made if needed. For example, your baby might do fine with yellow squash, but have a reaction to peas. Tummy discomfort, diarrhea, even rashes are common symptoms of food allergies and can also affect naps and nighttime sleep. Vomiting, while rare, is a more serious indicator that baby is having a reaction. The bottom line? Never introduce multiple food types at the same time so you will not have to guess which food caused the reaction, should one occur.

When introducing cereal into your baby's diet, begin with the morning meal. If, by any chance, your baby does have an intestinal reaction, it will be noticed and should be over by the end of the day. By starting a new food at noon or at dinner, you run the risk of pushing the reaction to the middle of the night when sleep disturbances are more difficult to discern.

Finally, before starting solids, check with immediate and extended family members to find out if there is a history of food allergies. Knowing whether allergies run in the family gives you a big advantage. If there is a history on either side, a higher probability exist that your little one will be challenged by food allergies. This is good information to have. If it happens, at least you are not caught off guard.

7. Baby is starting a sleep/nap transition because he is extending his nighttime sleep, affecting daytime naps.

Explanation/Recommendation: When a baby begins to extend his sleep at night, such as going from 10 to 12 hours, this naturally brings about a reduction in time the baby sleeps during the day. This reduction usually shows up at naptime (on rare occasions it can show up at 3:00 a.m., when baby wakes and wants to play). In this case, the baby is not adding or subtracting hours of sleep; he is rearranging when his sleep occurs. However, as Baby grows he will begin to subtract hours because his body will not allow him to over-sleep.

8. Baby is getting too much sleep and needs to subtract sleep hours.

Explanation/Recommendation: While sleep is very important to a baby's development and overall behavioral performance, there are limits to the amount of sleep a baby needs at each stage of growth. The "sleep-center" in a baby's brain will automatically begin to send an "awake signal" if there is too much sleep occurring in a 24-hour period. When he reaches this level of growth he will begin to subtract hours of sleep. Normally, babies do not subtract hours from nighttime sleep but from daytime sleep. Correspondingly, this means waketimes are extending, and the number of naps decrease during the day.

9. Baby is hungry because Mom's milk supply has gradually decreased.

Explanation/Recommendation: When it comes to a drop in

Mom's milk supply, the decrease is usually gradual, and correspondingly her baby gradually shifts nap duration. Baby might start waking just 15 to 30 minutes early, and then 30 to 45 minutes, or 60 minutes early. Most Moms can add a feeding or two and increase her milk supply.

However, there is a very small percentage of breastfeeding moms who are not able to sustain their milk supply during the day, even after trying every reasonable lactation suggestion offered. Sometimes, during the long stretch of nighttime sleep, Mom is able to produce a sufficient quantity of milk for the morning feed, but she is not able to sustain the necessary production throughout the day. The end result shows up at the various sleep times. Possible causes for lower milk production include:

- Mom is not offering enough feedings in a 24-hour period.
- Mom is fatigued because she is offering too many feedings (or is cluster-feeding).
- Mom's schedule is too busy (i.e. she is not getting sufficient rest).
- Mom is not eating properly or not taking in sufficient calories or liquids.
- Mom is on a lactation-suppressing medication.
- Mom is not able to keep up with baby's nutritional needs.

Once Mom discovers the probable cause for the decrease in her milk supply, she should take corrective action on any cause that she can control or influence. If she determines that she is not able to provide her baby adequate nutrition through exclusive breastfeeding, even after making all the proper nursing adjustments, then she has two choices. Continue to nurse and supplement with formula, or completely switch over to formula. Either way, the most important aspect is whether the baby is receiving adequate nutrition for healthy growth, and that is what Mom's decision should be based on.

10. Baby has a reaction to a new medication Mom is taking.

<u>Explanation/Recommendation</u>: Most medications prescribed to breastfeeding mothers are safe for the nursing infant. However, there are certain medications that can potentially become a source of discomfort, thereby impacting a baby's sleep. If Mom suspects a link between her medication and her baby's irritability, there are several factors to consider.

First, a mother should not assume that a medication safely taken during pregnancy will always be safe for a nursing baby. Second, Mom should check the prescription dosage with her doctor or pharmacist. Is it possible to reduce the dosage or substitute another drug that has less side effects for the baby? Third, what time of day is Mom taking her medication? Is it possible to take it right after baby's last feeding of the night, so her body can metabolize most of the medication during her nighttime sleep, which hopefully will be 8 to 10 hours before her baby's next meal? In the end, Mom must weigh the benefits of taking her medication in light of the possibility that the medication is having a negative impact on her baby. Getting advice from a medical expert should be considered.

11. An over-abundant milk supply is providing too much lactose for baby.

<u>Explanation/Recommendation</u>: Most breastfeeding concerns are associated with mothers who are not producing enough breastmilk. However, in rare cases, some mothers produce too much milk, which sets in motion a ripple effect that shows up at naptime. When a mother's milk-producing glands are making and storing more milk than her baby needs, then correspondingly, the foremilk/hindmilk volumes change. While the foremilk/hindmilk nutrient *ratios* remain the same, the total quantities in each breast are higher. When there is more foremilk available to a hungry baby, there is more lactose (milk sugar) ingested,

and that is when the problem starts.

Healthy babies do not have a problem with processing normal levels of lactose, but ingesting a large volume will overpower their digestive tracks because they do not have enough *lactase* (digestive enzyme) to break down all the lactose. Excessive lactose causes significant discomfort from gas build-up. Green watery stools are a common symptom of this condition.

Let's do the math on this. We will assume that Baby is at an age when he should be taking a total of 5 ounces of milk at each feeding, (2½ ounces from each breast). However, Mom is producing 6 to 8 ounces of milk at each feeding, which proportionally increases the amount of lactose available during nursing. Baby starts on one side, takes 3-4 ounces, switches breasts, but then becomes satiated with 2 ounces of mostly foremilk from the second side. Since foremilk is high in lactose but lower in fat than hindmilk, the result is too much lactose entering the baby's digestive system causing stomach pain, watery stools, and ultimately leading to disruptions at Baby's naptimes.

A downward cycle follows: naps become shorter, Baby begins to feed less vigorously and the lactose cycle repeats itself. Possible solution? Pumping some milk from both breast just prior to feeding might help remedy the problem. That will remove some of the foremilk so when Baby feeds, he will receive a closer to normal foremilk/hindmilk ratio. Unfortunately, trial and error is the only way to discover the right amount to pump.

12. Baby's waketime is too short.

<u>Explanation/Recommendation</u>: There will always be days when a baby's routine will have some variance impacting the length of waketimes. However, if a baby's waketime is routinely too short for his age, then naptimes will be disrupted

13. Baby's waketimes are over-stimulating or too long.

<u>Explanation/Recommendation</u>: When searching for the solution

to naptime challenges, parents often overlook the quality of the waketime that preceded the nap. Remember, everything is connected. Waketimes affect naps just like naps affect waketimes. Over-tired and over-stimulated babies become hyper-alert, fighting off sleep through crying. If this is a regular problem, shortening your baby's waketime by 15-minute increments might help.

Also, be aware of the types of activities you and your baby are involved in. Are you having too many visitors drop by who have an irresistible urge to entertain your baby? Was your baby being exposed to Dad's loud friends as they sat watching a sporting event? Might Mom be on the go too much? When Baby is along for the ride, the coming and going, the new sights and sounds, and the absence of predictability all work against good nap behavior. That is because catnaps in a car seat are no substitute for a full nap in the crib. An occasional nap in the car seat will not cause trouble, but it should not be the norm, especially during the first six months of your baby's life.

14. First feeding of the day has too much flexibility.

Explanation/Recommendation: As previously noted, it is important that the first feeding of the day stays fairly consistent (within 20 to 30 minutes.) Otherwise, each day will be a different rhythm, which works against stabilizing the baby's hunger metabolism. This will eventually affect the length of baby's naptime.

15. Baby is not being exposed to adequate amounts of daylight.

Explanation/Recommendation: Natural light is important to help babies regulate their circadian clock. This is the inner clock, the biological time-keeping system that regulates daily activities, such as sleep and wake cycles. We recommend that, as soon as your baby awakens in the morning, you take him to a room filled with daylight (although he does not need to be in direct sunlight). Natural light, along with the first feeding of the day, will help establish his circadian rhythm and keep them consistent. Routine helps facilitate this amazing function possessed by all humans.

16. Baby's room is not dark enough.

Explanation/Recommendation: This is one of the most overlooked reasons for a sudden occurrence of baby waking early and one of the easiest to fix. While newborns can sleep just about anywhere and under any conditions, the "light sensitivity" begins to change after three months of age. The morning sun is on one side of the house, but the afternoon sun is on another. Depending on the direction that the baby's room faces, the sun's light can impact a baby's naps. Like most adults, babies tend to sleep better and longer if the room is darkened. Shades or curtains are the simple solution.

17. Baby is over-stimulated in the crib because a wind-up toy/mobile was turned on when he was put down for a nap.

Explanation/Recommendation: All those fun baby gifts Mom and Dad want to use right away can be a problem. Why? Newborns are not ready to appreciate crib gear yet because of their eyesight. Prior to four months of age, we recommend keeping the crib mobiles in their boxes. When they come out, put them over the playpen rather than the crib. Mobiles are entertaining, but when set up too early and activated just before naptime, they can become a source of over-stimulation. Some babies cannot neurologically handle particular types of stimulation created by movement and sound. Even the flickering of light from a television can over-stimulate a baby.

For example, Mom is checking her social media feeds, in a darkened room, while nursing and notices her baby drifting off to sleep. She thinks he must be tired, however, in this case the baby is shutting down neurologically, a mechanism by which a baby's body protects itself. Thirty minutes later, the baby wakes and Mom interprets this as a sleep problem, when it is actually a problem brought on by over-stimulation. The problem here is the "blue-light" emitting from her phone screen, disrupts the production of *melatonin,* which is necessary for establishing and maintaining natural sleep-wake cycles. The "blue-light" is not only effecting Baby, but Mom's ability to sleep well.

18. Your four to six-month-old baby is waking in response to sounds associated with pleasure.

Explanation/Recommendation: This condition is created when two time-elements cross. The baby's circadian clock has him moving out of deep sleep into active sleep close to the time a familiar sound occurs each day. As he approaches four months, he develops the ability to associate sounds with activities and people. Once he makes the association, he becomes more alert and the sound can trigger an awake mode. While many babies will fall back to sleep, others are ready to fight off sleep in exchange for the next big adventure.

It could be the familiar sound of school-bus brakes or a garage-door opening. Both signal the arrival of someone, perhaps an entertaining sibling or fun-loving Dad. There is very little you can do about the school-bus brakes except to substitute some white noise during the naptime affected. Dad can park the car in the driveway, and find a less disturbing way to enter the house. Every home has its own peculiar sounds that become part of a baby's subconscious, especially if the sound precedes pleasure. It is as if a bell goes off in Baby's head and suddenly he is ready to party!

19. Unknown: What does this mean? Simply that a reason exists, but it is so unique to your baby's situation that it is not easily duplicated by other babies.

<u>Explanation/Recommendation</u>: It is both amazing and helpful to realize that the simplest things can get overlooked when searching for a sleep/nap solution. One mother reported her search ended when she went into her baby's room, after he fell asleep, and started sitting through his nap. She was not sure what she was looking for, but she discovered something she never expected. Just about 35 minutes into his nap, a beam of sunlight shining down onto her baby's face began to appear. In this case, the unknown factor was tied to the earth's rotation, which continually changed the angle of the sun. In tracing the sunbeam back to its source, Mom discovered the sun's rays were reflecting off a piece of metal flashing on her neighbor's roof. While the sun's impact at that exact location lasted only ten minutes, it was enough to wake the baby. Mom hung a towel in the corner of the window during naptime and that solved the problem.

If the cause of your baby's naptime disturbance falls into the category of "unknown," Keep looking for clues, ask questions, or invite an experienced *PDF* mom over for part of the day to observe you and your baby. If stumped with a nap challenge, a fresh set of eyes can never hurt.

SUMMARY OF WAKING EARLY

If your baby wakes early out of a sound sleep with a strong cry, consider whether the cause relates to Baby, Mom, waketime, or the sleep environment. This phenomenon has become known as the 45-Minute Intruder and can visit your baby at anytime; but it usually shows up after eight weeks of age and peaks around six months of age. It might stick around a day or two or decide to take up residence for a week.

If you have ruled out the simple explanations, we suggest you begin by treating the sleep intruder as a hunger problem. Try feeding your baby first. If he shows no interest in feeding or does not feed well, you have just ruled out hunger as the cause. But if he does take a full feeding, you have narrowed the problem to a feeding issue. This could be an indicator that he is starting a growth spurt, or there is a decrease in your milk supply or the quality of your milk.

If this is not a feeding issue, then go through the rest of the items in List Two. The key to fixing the problem is to identify the source of the problem and then work toward a solution. Even if you cannot identify the source, the problem tends to be temporary and usually fixes itself.

Finally, be aware that some sleep advocates advise moms to keep their babies on fixed schedules, even if their babies wake early from their naps. Their advice is to allow the baby to "cry it out" until the next feeding, but this ignores the potential needs of the baby. *A hungry baby should always be fed!* Withholding food is never a way to fix a sleep problem.

SUMMARY: WAKETIME AND NAPS

Waketime will become an increasingly important part of your baby's day, because it is a time of learning. There is a balance however, that parents must stay mindful of. Over-stimulating a baby during waketime impacts the next set of feedings and naptimes. Remember, everything is connected.

When parents help their babies by establishing healthy feed-wake-sleep patterns, everyone in the house wins. When there are a number of disruptions in your baby's feeding or waketime routine, there will be corresponding changes in his sleep patterns. Stay on top of this by being as consistent as possible with mealtime and age-appropriate waketimes. There are more developmental resources online to help you make the most of your baby's waketimes and naps. Connect with other new moms at *www.Facebook.com/BabywiseLife*.

Chapter Seven

When Your Baby Cries

Your baby cries and the world around you goes dim. You know a message is in there somewhere—but what is it? Besides crying when hungry, babies have their own way of singing the blues when tired, wet, sick, bored, frustrated, out of their routine, or fed too often; sometimes it is simply because that is what normal, healthy babies do. No parent finds pleasure in hearing that sound, especially if you are a first-time parent. A baby's cry evokes feelings of uncertainty unlike anything experienced before. It is a powerful, uncomfortable sensation that makes mothers and father wonder if they overlooked or did something wrong, and this can often lead to anxious moments. If you only knew what to do! We trust, after reading this chapter, you will.

To begin with, it is reassuring to know that the American Academy of Pediatrics recognizes crying as a natural part of a baby's day. From their complete and authoritative guide for infant care, we read: "All babies cry, often without any apparent cause. Newborns routinely cry a total of 1 to 4 hours a day. No mother can console her child every time he cries, so do not expect to be a miracle worker with your baby. Pay close attention to your baby's different cries and you'll soon be able to tell when he needs to be picked up, consoled, or tended to, and when he is better off left alone."(1)

Think of crying as a signal, not a statement against your parenting. As a mom or dad, learn to assess your baby's cry, so you can respond properly. The ability to *read* your baby's cry will give you confidence in parenting, but what are the keys to decoding Baby's signal?

In early infancy, crying is an intuitive way of communicating both need and displeasure. The hunger cry is different from the sick cry. The sleepy cry is different from the "cuddle me" cry. And the distress cry differs from the demanding cry. Crying varies in volume, too. Sometimes a cry will be nothing more than a gentle whimper. Other times it is a violent protest. Be aware that attempts to minimize or "block" all crying can easily increase your baby's stress (and yours) rather than decrease it. It has been well documented that tears shed from crying help to eliminate chemically activated stress hormones from the body.

THE INEVITABLE CONFLICT

In the world of babyhood advice, there are two fringe groups to avoid: the "Let Baby cry it out" group and the "Block every cry" advocates. Advice from either is not helpful because it requires parents to surrender their common sense to extreme beliefs. The first comes from the Behaviorist movement described in Chapter Two. With them, the end (a well-scheduled child) justifies the means. But what about legitimate hunger cues that come sooner than a scheduled feeding? With strict Clock Feeding, a baby is left to cry, often needlessly. At the other extreme is Attachment Parenting, which promotes blocking or suppressing all crying, driven by the false assumption that a baby's cry reflects the anxiety left over from the supposed trauma sustained at birth.

Some interesting research demonstrated that infants who were allowed to cry during the normal times in infancy were vigorous and active problem solvers at one year of age. When presented with obstacles separating them from their parents, they found a way to maneuver around the barriers to get back to Mom or Dad. They were neither stressed nor frightened. In contrast, the babies whose parents routinely suppressed their cries could not overcome the simplest obstacles separating them from their parents. They tended to sit, whimper and wait to be rescued. They lost all sense of initiative to help themselves.[2]

What might this prove? When crying is suppressed, rather than managing the moment according to the need, infants learn to rely on crying for all their problem solving. When parents block their baby's every cry rather than manage it according to the baby's need, they are inadvertently closing off in their baby's mind other vital associations. For example, infants learn very quickly that an action is usually followed by a predictable response. If Baby is hungry and cries, feeding usually follows. If he soils his diaper, changing takes place. If he is startled, he is comforted. If placed in his crib, he learns that sleep comes next. Such learning association provides the building blocks for complex skills, including soothing oneself and problem solving. When parents attempt to suppress all crying, they deny their baby access to the learning patterns that come with association.

UNDERSTANDING YOUR BABY'S CRY

The key to understanding and properly responding to a baby's cry is assessing the context of the crying, not just the cry itself. There are six specific cry times during the first five months of life: Three of them are *abnormal* cry periods: three are *normal* periods. The abnormal cries signal that something is wrong and should be checked. The normal cries are still signals, but call for different responses. Here is the breakdown of each.

Abnormal Crying

Crying during feedings, immediately after feedings and in the middle of a sound nap require attention, because these are not times when a baby should be crying. Do not wait for the crying to subside; investigate and look for the root cause.

<u>Crying During Feeding</u>: This is not normal. Is the baby frustrated or overwhelmed? Is the milk coming too fast or not fast enough? There could be a number of reasons for these condi-

tions, including improper latching on or poor milk release. (See Appendix Four, Monitoring Your Baby's Growth).

Crying Immediately after Feeding: If your baby cries routinely within 30 minutes after feeding, and it sounds more like a cry from pain than sleepiness, it may be caused by one of several factors:

1. Trapped gas. Young babies often swallow air during feedings. This air must be brought up again. Burp your baby by holding him against your shoulder, on your lap or over your knee (as shown in Chapter Four). Trapped gas is the first cause to consider when a baby wakes up 30 minutes into a nap. This cry is often a high-pitched scream. If that is your situation, pick the baby up, try burping and cuddling for a moment, and then put the baby back down.
2. Mom's diet. If crying after a feeding is a problem, it might be helpful to keep a record of the foods eaten just before each nursing session, and measure your baby's response based on what foods you are eliminating or cutting back on. Stay mindful of dairy products and spicy/gas producing foods. They are a leading cause of a baby's digestive discomfort.
3. A milk-quality problem. A breastfeeding mother can have a sufficient quantity of milk, but not sufficient quality. If that is the problem, the baby will respond with a hunger cry/cue within an hour. Although this condition is rare, it may affect as many as five percent of nursing mothers. What can you do to improve this condition? Check your diet and seek your pediatrician's counsel. He or she may recommend a nutritionist.

Crying in the Middle of a Sound Nap: If your baby wakes out of a sound sleep with a strong cry, it may be from a combination of any of the three factors mentioned above. It may be that his sleep schedule was disrupted from a previous late evening or hectic morning. It may also be one of the multiple factors noted in Chapter Six relating to nap challenges. For example, if your baby demonstrates a need to feed more often by waking out of a sound nap, it may indicate a decrease in your milk supply or the quality of your milk. By all means, feed your baby, but do not stop there. Try to find out why your baby is suddenly showing signs of hunger. By feeding sooner than normal, you are not going backward in your routine, but are making a healthy and proper adjustment to moving forward into the next phase of your baby's development.

Normal Crying

Except the ones just mentioned, other types of crying are normal and should be expected. These include crying just before feeding, during the late-afternoon/early-evening period and when Baby is put down for a nap or to sleep for the night.

<u>Crying Just before Feeding.</u> Under normal circumstances, this kind of crying is very short, since the next event for the baby is mealtime. If your baby is hungry, feed him. If he routinely shows signs of hunger before the next scheduled feeding, find out why, rather than letting him cry it out. Your baby's routine is to serve you and your baby, not the reverse.

<u>Crying During the Late-Afternoon/Early-Evening Period</u>. Most babies have a "personal fussy time," especially in the late afternoon. That is true of both bottle and breastfed infants, and you are in good company: literally millions of mothers and fathers are going through the same thing at nearly the same time as you each day.

If your fussy baby is not comforted by the baby swing, an infant seat, siblings or Grandma, consider the crib. At least there he has the chance of falling asleep and putting everyone out of this temporary misery. If you have a baby who becomes exceptionally and continuously fussy, consider the possibility that he is hungry. How is your milk supply? How is your diet?

The challenges of crying associated with colic and reflux are taken up in our next chapter.

Crying When Going Down for a Nap. When your baby goes down for a nap, the duration of crying is set by the child but monitored by the parent. Crying for some children seems to be an art form, despite the fact that he is nurtured, loved and cared for with great devotion and intensity. Some babies have a greater propensity to cry, especially when being put down for a nap. This is not a signal that their basic needs are not being met, but that some babies have a disposition to cry that we wish they did not have! The American Academy of Pediatrics recognizes this fact: "Many babies cannot fall asleep without crying and will go to sleep more quickly if left to cry for a while. The crying should not last long if the child is truly tired."[3]

It is not unusual for a sleeping baby occasionally to whimper or cry softly in the middle of a nap. Again, the words of the AAP are helpful in understanding what might be going on: "Sometimes you may think your baby is waking up when he is actually going through a phase of very light slumber. He could be startled, squirming, fussing, or even crying—and still be asleep. Or he may be awake but on the verge of drifting off again if left alone. Do not make the mistake of trying to comfort him during these moments; you will only awaken him further and delay him from going back to sleep. Instead, if you let him fuss and even cry for a few minutes, he will learn to get himself to sleep without relying on you."[4]

The Academy goes on to say that "some babies actually need to let off energy by crying in order to settle into sleep or rouse themselves out of it. As much as fifteen to twenty minutes of fussing will not do your child any harm. Just be sure he is not crying out of hunger or pain, or because his diaper is wet."[5]

With the goal of teaching good sleep habits, some temporary crying is preferable over poor sleep habits that are far more harmful than a little crying. The benefits of healthy sleep training come early. Expect a well-rested baby to be a good feeder. Also, you can put your baby down for his nap or bedtime and walk away. The child falls right to sleep and wakes with contentment. Another advantage to this sleep training is that you may put your baby down at anyone's house and have the same success.

Some babies cry 15 minutes before falling asleep. Others vary the duration of their cry from five minutes at one naptime to an off-and-on 35-minute cry at another. If your baby cries longer than 15 minutes, check on him. Pat him on the back and possibly hold him for a moment. Then put him back down. Remember, you are not training your baby not to cry, but how to sleep. This may be the only time in your baby's day when the practice of non-intervention is best.

Identifying Cry Patterns

Identifying and knowing your baby's cry patterns and disposition or personal style will help you discern real needs. Some babies have a naptime cry pattern like a bell curve: a gentle whimper built to a mild wail, which then falls back again to a whimper. Sleep follows. The total time elapsed might be 10 to 15 minutes. A second pattern has a baby crying ten minutes, then stopping, then a minute later starting again for five more minutes, followed by sleep.

A third baby provides yet another pattern. The Ezzos have a granddaughter whose infant cry climbed rapidly from a whimper to a wail. Then at the height of her cry, she would stop abruptly and drop off to a sound sleep. After the first month, a change in her cry duration became apparent; times averaged five to ten minutes in length. Eventually she became selective as to which naptimes to cry. After three months, however, crying at naptime became rare, while healthy, continuous nap and nighttime sleep became the norm.

Become a student of your baby's cry patterns When you do, you will know what is normal for him. He may be selective about which naptime he cries, but if you are patient and understanding, healthy naps and nighttime sleep will be the great reward.

Cries to Listen For

As we stated previously, some crying is normal and as a parent, you should expect it. However, you also need to stay alert to certain identifiable cries. For example, a high-pitched, piercing cry may be a signal of either internal or external bodily injury. Such a cry, if persistent, should be brought to the attention of your pediatrician.

A marked change in your baby's crying pattern may be a warning of illness. Look for a sudden increase in the frequency and duration of crying or a weak, mousy cry. Discuss this with your pediatrician. Cries indicating hunger or thirst are predictable with *PDF* babies. You can be certain the cry is not a hunger-and-thirst cry, if your baby is satisfied after a feeding. With demand-fed babies, their cries are unpredictable, leaving Mom and Dad guessing and anxious.

Babies who routinely cry and act hungry after only 1½ hours are probably not getting enough food. If you are breastfeeding, check your milk supply and the factors that influence it. If your baby wakes up in the middle of a nap with a loud, piercing cry, be sure to investigate. This could be caused by gas buildup or something in your breastmilk as a result of something you ate earlier in the day. If this cry persists, physically check your baby.

RESPONDING TO YOUR BABY'S CRY

How long should you let your baby cry? Respond immediately to abnormal crying, however, some cries should be guided by the following suggestions.

1. Think about Where Your Baby Is in His Routine: Is naptime finished, or is he in the middle of his nap, needing to resettle? Does he need to go down for a nap? Has he been in the swing

too long? Did he lose his toy? Did he spit up? Is this his fussy time of day? This is only a short list of why your baby might be crying. There are many reasons other than hunger that can cause him to turn on the tears, and they are all legitimate reasons. First determine the cause, then respond appropriately.

2. Listen for the Type of Cry: Even in the early days and weeks, you will begin to distinguish different tones and patterns in your baby's crying. Simply stop and listen. You may find that the crying ends as quickly as it began, especially during naptime. By listening you can determine a right response.

3. Take Action: Just remember, sometimes the best action is no action at all. For example, if your baby is clean, fed, and ready for naptime, let him learn how to fall asleep alone. This may be precisely what your baby needs. If you get into the habit of nursing him to sleep, then you have only succeeded in creating a sleep prop. That will not help the baby.

If he cries, take note of how long it lasts. Moms are often surprised to learn that the seemingly endless bout of crying lasted only a few minutes. In the event that you have listened, waited and determined that the crying is not subsiding, gather more information by checking on the baby. Peek into his crib and see if he has become jammed into a corner. If so, simply move him and offer a gentle pat on the back before leaving the room.

There will be times when your assessment calls for picking up and holding your baby, even if it is only to reassure him that everything is all right. Sometimes there is no rhyme or reason behind the need for special time in Mommy's arms. The point is this: your assessment may produce many options, but blocking your child's cry all the time because you cannot handle the sound of the cry should not be one of them.

When Should I Hold and Comfort My Baby?

You will, of course, hold your baby many hours each day.

As you care for and feed your baby, holding and cuddling him comes naturally. Flirt with Baby. Rock him in your arms. Sing a sweet song to him. Happy or not so happy, Baby loves the attention. Wouldn't you? Realize, however, it is easy to overdo the attention when your baby is fussy.

Parents should offer comfort when comfort is needed, but stay mindful of what type of comfort is actually needed? A diaper change will comfort a wet baby. A feeding will comfort a hungry baby. Holding will comfort a startled baby, and sleep will comfort a tired baby. A baby can receive comfort in many other ways, such as being rocked, sung to, taken for a stroller ride and being near a source of music. That comfort can come from different people. Certainly Dad, older siblings, Grandma and Grandpa can be great sources of comfort.

Wisdom dictates that a mother should recognize that a baby responds to different forms of comfort at different times. If you use one source exclusively, such as nursing, you are not necessarily comforting your baby, only stopping his cry by arousing the sucking reflex. If nursing is the only form of comfort, other real needs will go unmet

SUMMARY

As a parent, learn to recognize your baby's different cries—listen, think and then take action. Remember that as your baby grows, his patterns of crying may change. He may be fed, clean, dry, and healthy when one day he begins to cry before falling asleep. Just consider that one more phase of your child's normal development.

Connect online with other like-minded moms at <u>www.Facebook.com/BabywiseLife</u>.

Chapter Eight

Colic, Reflux and the Inconsolable Baby

When a mother and father behold the wonder of a new life, they can easily feel overwhelmed. There is so much to learn about raising a child, and so much pressure when starting out with a newborn. But there is some encouraging news. A *Babywise* routine can settle much of a parent's anxiety since it brings order to a baby's life, and as a result, that brings confidence to a parent's heart.

Yet, we all know that life is not always predictable. What happens when a baby does not follow the routine and shows signs of fussiness beyond the normal times? Perhaps he cries for food, but a few minutes into his feeding he stops and refuses to nurse or take his bottle. Maybe he arches his back in pain but rejects your comforting efforts. Or, scarier, he spits up what looks like his entire meal at every meal, in addition to waking out of a sound nap and crying in discomfort. What should you do?

In the previous chapter we contrasted normal and abnormal cry periods. Some babies cry before a feeding or when going down for a nap. They have a fussy time at least once a day, often in the late afternoon, but are usually in a relatively peaceful condition the rest of the day. These are the normal, even expected fussy times common during infancy.

However, what about parents who have a son like Asher or Ross, who showed all the signs of hunger, latched on to Mom, started feeding and then after a few minutes stopped cold. Once they started crying they recoiled from nursing any longer. Out of exhaustion they fell asleep, but 30 minutes later woke up hungry and the frustrating cycle repeated itself. Or maybe they have a son like Caleb who was inconsolable and fussed all the time, screaming before, during, and after feedings, pulling up his little legs in abdominal pain. Other parents have an infant like little Micah, who vomited every meal for six months. For these parents, the cause of their baby's discomfort was baffling, blending desperation and fatigue with the agony of concern. Here are a few more details.

ASHER'S STORY

According to Ashley, Asher's mom, it happened at every feeding:

"Asher showed all the normal hunger signals, began to nurse ferociously, and then would suddenly stop. He would pull away from me and just start screaming. I knew something was wrong, but what? I tried everything. I changed my diet, fed more often, fed less often, switched sides numerous times while nursing, and burped him often. Nothing helped. Sleep was not the best. Asher took very short naps, 30 minutes, if I could get him to sleep at all. At night he would wake four to five times. Nothing brought comfort to my son."

MICAH'S STORY

Whitney provided a slightly different account of her son, Micah, but one just as stressful:

"Forester, my firstborn, was a big spitter (soaked a burp cloth every feeding), but he was a happy spitter and a big baby (9 lbs. 11 oz. at birth). He remained at the top of the growth charts, so I never thought twice about colic or reflux. After my second child, Micah, was born, I saw a similar pattern developing. By his second day of life, Micah was spitting up large amounts after each feed. At first I just thought he was a big spitter like my firstborn, but by the end of Micah's first week, my husband said, 'This just cannot be normal.' At two weeks Micah was spitting up 40-50 times a day. There were times when he spit up so much milk that I would wonder if I should feed him again because it looked like everything just came back up.

He remained on a 2-hour feeding routine for the first three months which wreaked havoc on his sleep cycles, and mine! I was discouraged and anxious. I remember being totally exhausted one night, crying at 2:00 a.m., thinking, 'I'm never going to rest, and he is never going to sleep! By the time he stops spitting up, it is time to feed again, and we are going to start all over!' I now realize that my first son, Forester, probably had a similar condition as a newborn."

ROSS'S STORY

Sally, Ross's mom, recalls:

"From the very beginning, we discovered that Ross had a pattern of spitting up during and after each meal. At three weeks, we noticed Ross had difficulty nursing and pulled off me and began crying during feedings. To say the least, feeding became a traumatic event for us both, as Ross would continually pull off, arch his back and cry, try to suck, and then pull off again. Although he slept fairly well, he was still waking at 3:00 a.m. or so at three months of age and had only moderate weight gain."

CALEB'S STORY

Caleb's struggles were even more distressing His mom, Stephanie, writes:

"Although I had a C-section when Caleb was born, he was very healthy and weighed in at six and one-half pounds. Initially, he was cast as an "easy" baby. He nursed well, had a ravenous appetite and those first few naps were wonderful. But my peaceful assessment and my easy-going baby lasted only a few days.

"By the end of the first week, everything started going downhill and fast! Caleb was very fussy and always seemed to be in pain and distress. If I was lucky, he would sleep for an hour and a half at a stretch, but then he would wake up screaming, covered in vomit. At his two-week checkup, Caleb was weighed and measured, and I was told he was growing beautifully. He had grown from six and one-half pounds at birth to nine pounds. I relayed all of the problems Caleb was having to the doctor, but I was assured it was 'just colic and a little bit of reflux.' When I tried to insist it was more, I was told there was nothing to worry about because he was gaining weight beautifully.

"Of course, everything was not fine. Caleb's condition grew worse. During feedings he would arch his back and be as stiff as a board. Caleb kept his legs drawn up to his stomach and his arms clenched tightly to his sides. Changing, dressing, and bathing him were a chore due to his stiffness. His condition necessitated a visit to a gastroenterologist. After taking Caleb's history, the gastroenterologist examined him and did an ultrasound of his abdomen. Based on the findings, he said that Caleb had a severe case of gastroesophageal reflux disease (GERD)."

This chapter addresses three medical conditions. While each condition has its own diagnosis, they are related symptomatically through crying and spitting up. The three conditions are:

1. Colic
2. Gastroesophageal reflux (GER)
3. Gastroesophageal reflux disease (GERD)

We hope that by alerting you to the conditions from which these four baby boys suffered, you will be proactive in seeking immediate medical attention should your baby demonstrate any of the distress signs. With Asher, Micah, Ross, and Caleb, all four were gaining weight, but that did not mean everything was medically okay with them. No one knows a baby like his parents, and if you sense something is not right, for your own peace of mind and your baby's health, pursue medical advice until you are satisfied your baby's condition is understood.

CRYING AND COLIC

There is a big difference between a fussy baby and a colicky baby. Fussy babies have fussy times followed by relative peace and calm the rest of the day or night. The colicky baby seems irritable nearly all the time, day and night. Symptoms of colic include piercing cries combined with these signs of acute stomach distress: folding of the legs, flailing arms, inconsolable crying and passing gas. Although this list of symptoms makes colic sound like a digestive disorder, it is not.

Most theorists suggest that colic is the immaturity of a baby's nervous system in being able to process the full range of stimuli common among newborns at birth. This condition affects about 20 percent of the infant population. It shows up usually between weeks two to four and generally ends by the third month. While there are no significant medical concerns associated with "true colic," a term that indicates how easily the condition can be misdiagnosed, the main problem is the stress and anxiety it creates within the home. It is emotionally difficult to cope with the constant crying of an inconsolable baby. Close friends and extended family can really help by giving the frazzled parents short breaks during this temporary crisis.

WHAT CAN A MOTHER DO?

It would be wonderful if there were a medical cure for colic or some homespun remedy that could bring babies relief from their physical distress. However, to date, no such cure exist. But there is some encouraging news. Colic, while distressing to parents, is not hopeless, and babies do outgrow it. If your baby is showing signs of colic, here are some practical suggestions from some of our experienced mothers of colic babies.

1. Always consult your pediatrician to rule out any medical reasons for your baby's excessive crying or spitting up. Ask your practitioner what might be helpful for your infant. Get a second opinion, if you sense your concerns are not being taken seriously.

2. Remember that all babies are different and respond to different measures. Find out what works for your baby and stay with it. Some moms have found it helpful to wrap their newborns in swaddling cloths, while others find giving a warm bath helpful or placing the infant in a swing or near a vibrating dryer (not on the dryer). If you are bottle feeding your baby, try changing formula. Your pediatrician can advise you.

3. A breastfeeding mom may find that certain foods in her diet trigger Baby's discomfort. You can start by eliminating gas-producing foods (e.g., beans, broccoli, cauliflower, cabbage, onions and garlic) or any spicy foods, then dairy products, caffeine and alcohol. Be systematic so you can identify a particular food or type of food that may be causing problems for your baby. If food sensitivity is the issue, there will be a noticeable decrease in your baby's colic-like symptoms within a couple of days. After a few weeks, gradually reintroduce individual items back into your diet and watch for a reaction.

4. Avoid having your baby around secondhand smoke, especially when you have colic symptoms to deal with.

5. It may help to give your baby a pacifier, especially after a feeding. Pacifiers bring comfort and help babies relax, although some babies show no interest in them. (Some research suggests that SIDS rates among infants who use a pacifier is significantly lower that those who do not.)

6. Colicky babies need to be burped frequently. If you are bottle feeding, try a different bottle or nipple designed to help reduce the amount of air your baby swallows during a feeding. Some of the bottles made for this purpose are curved, vented, or have a collapsible bag inside. After each feeding, lay your baby across your knees, stomach down, and gently massage his back. The pressure of your knees against his abdomen may help relieve his discomfort.

7. Most newborns, especially those struggling with colic, have a low threshold for rapid movements, such as the flickering of a computer screen. A baby's developing neurological system has difficulty processing rapid light and sound changes. Such stimulation may further heighten an already stressful situation. Try offering your feedings in a soothing, calming environment.

8. At the other end of the spectrum are babies who are comforted by rhythmic motion, steady sound (commonly called white noise) or both. Some parents find securely placing their infant in the baby swing close to the 'white noise provides some temporary relief.

TAKING CARE OF YOU

First-time moms and dads may find the early months of parenthood challenging beyond belief, especially if they have a colicky baby. One of the best things you can do for your baby is to take care of yourself. As much as reasonable, keep your baby's routine going, but if you are feeling overwhelmed, take a break. Ask a family member or friend to take over for a while, even if it is only for an hour or two. While time seems to move slowly during stressful situations, keep in mind this hope-giving truth: your baby will outgrow his colic and life will return to normal.

REFLUX AND GERD

One of the biggest medical risks associated with colic is not the condition itself, but its symptoms because they mimic and often mask serious conditions such as milk-protein allergies, lactose intolerance, gastroesophageal reflux (GER), and gastroesophageal reflux disease (GERD).

GERD is a serious digestive problem in newborns that is often missed because it is too quickly labeled as colic. It is not the same as GER (gastroesophageal reflux) or just plain reflux. *GER causes asymptomatic spitting up* and does not require medical treatment because the baby is growing well and is not fussy. *GERD, however, causes intense pain and will lead to a feeding aversion if not treated.* Caleb's case manifested pain, inconsolable crying and excessive spitting up although his weight gain was excellent; so it took awhile to diagnose the true condition. GERD requires medical attention, usually in the form of medication to decrease gastric-acid production; but it sometimes calls for surgical repair. The encouraging news is this condition is highly manageable.

REFLUX/GERD: WHAT DO WE KNOW?

Note: For purposes of this discussion, the term, "Reflux," applies to both GER and GERD. Approximately 2½ million babies are born every day around the world, and many will experience a minor degree of reflux. This reflux decreases as the newborn's digestive system matures. It is estimated that in the United States, three to five percent of all newborns have mild to severe reflux symptoms for the first few months of life. *Reflux is usually due to an immature sphincter valve between the stomach and the esophagus.* When working properly, the valve opens to allow us to swallow, burp or vomit and closes immediately afterward. Reflux occurs when the sphincter either stays relaxed or relaxes periodically, allowing food mixed with stomach acid to back up into the esophagus and throat, causing a burning sensation.

Reflux usually presents itself in the first few weeks of life. It often corrects itself, but in extreme cases, the infant may develop a feeding aversion because he associates feeding with pain. The condition can advance to the point where it causes significant weight loss or *esophagitis*, creating a condition known as "failure to thrive." When reflux requires advanced medical attention beyond observation, the baby is said to have *GERD*.

Many babies with reflux are happy and thriving, despite their excessive spitting up. These little ones are sometimes called "happy spitters" or "happy chuckers," and require little medical intervention. They are growing well, are not abnormally fussy and not in significant pain. They usually outgrow their reflux without complications. A smaller percentage of babies, however, like Asher, Micah, Ross, and Caleb, suffer with a type of severe infantile heartburn that requires medical attention. These are the GERD babies.

One of the most important indicators of GERD is an infant's inability to be consoled. He is crying because he is in pain. If GERD is the issue, when a physician prescribes a medication that blocks acid production in the stomach, you will see some improvement within two days and substantial improvement within 14 days. If no improvement takes place, the parents need to contact their healthcare provider immediately to find what will help their baby.

There are a number of diagnostic tests available to confirm the diagnosis of GERD. Your baby's symptoms will direct the doctor in determining which test will be most appropriate. If you are not comfortable with or do not understand the pros and cons of the prescribed treatment or tests, request a second opinion. Dealing with any form of reflux is emotionally stressful for parents. You must have confidence and understanding, so that you can wisely cooperate with your baby's healthcare provider and together bring relief and soothing comfort to your baby.

In addition to medication, there are aggravating food-source considerations for breastfeeding moms to review. Proper feeding positioning for the baby is important. Holding a baby at a 30-degree angle (the most natural angle for breast or bottle-fed infants) will result in fewer reflux episodes than when a baby is held horizontally.

COLIC, REFLUX, AND THE *BABYWISE PDF* ROUTINE

Parents who have an infant with either colic or reflux (GER or GERD) may assume the *PDF* routine will not work for them, but the opposite is true. *Babywise* will help you recognize progress and bring order to an otherwise chaotic situation. Although you may need to make adaptations to the *PDF* routine for your unique situation, you are still providing what is best for your baby and managing his particular needs. Let's now consider how colic and reflux issues affect feedings, waketimes, and sleeping.

Challenges with the Routine

1. In general, try to keep your baby on a regular routine. With a reflux baby, consider feeding more often than the 2½ to 3 hours generally recommended (possibly every 2 hours). This may be easier on your baby since he will not try to get as much food each time. The pressure of a full stomach could worsen his reflux. Use routinely whatever time increment you find helpful to your baby.

2. The basic principles of *Babywise* remain the same, including the establishment of healthy feed, wake, and sleep cycles. A well-established sleep pattern can take longer to accomplish with reflux, but it will come. In Asher's case, consistent, uninterrupted nighttime sleep was not achieved until he was six months old. It should be noted however, that some reflux

babies begin sleeping through the night between 13-18 weeks.

3. Keep Baby's environment calm and quiet. Try wrapping him snuggly to minimize extra stimulation and stress. Hold him gently and avoid bouncing, jiggling or excessive back patting.

4. Do not worry that your baby is not following the plan exactly like the book describes. Instead, learn to enjoy his uniqueness in spite of your baby's digestive condition.

Feeding Times/Waketimes

1. As a parent, avoid the two feeding extremes: letting your baby get too hungry and over-feeding him.

2. Keep the feeding environment calm and relaxing. Turn off the television and any loud music (carries vibrations that some newborns find irritating).

3. Try propping your baby in an upright position after each feeding for at least 30 minutes or elevating his crib mattress slightly (maximum of 30 degrees). This will help with digestion Also remember, be sure to burp him frequently.

4. If a particular feeding is dragging out longer than 45 minutes, either because he no longer seems interested, or is struggling due to discomfort, discontinue the feeding, burp well and then use recommendation of #3 above. It is better to let him wake earlier (but hungry) at his next feeding than to go at it for an hour just to get a full feeding. This will only exhaust parent and child.

5. Some breastfeeding mothers have an overflowing supply of milk. Their babies will attempt to compensate by swallowing faster and gulping, taking in excessive air, which produces gas. That exacerbates the reflux condition. If this is your situation,

allow gravity to help solve the problem. Either recline in a lounge chair or lie down propped on a pillow (so you are not completely reclining), and gravity will slow down the force of your letdown.

Another technique is to use your index and middle fingers for a gentle scissors hold to control the initial flow of milk during your letdown. When your letdown begins, direct the initial spray into a towel and then bring your baby back to your breast.

6. For babies diagnosed with reflux and spit up, the AAP suggests hold off offering an additional feed and instead wait until the next feeding.

7. It is sometimes suggested that bottle-fed babies who suffer from reflux may benefit from having their formula thickened with rice cereal (usually one tablespoon per one ounce of formula. Here again, check with your pediatrician first)

8. If your pediatrician recommends any medicine for your baby, ask about the possible side effects. Some medications can give babies stomach cramps, which may appear as colic.

9. When changing your baby, take care not to pull the diaper too tight. That can place additional pressure on his stomach.

Sleeping

Sleep can seem impossible when a baby is waking up screaming 35 to 45 minutes into his sleep cycle. Here are some practical suggestions to consider.

1. You might try swaddling your baby when putting him down for a nap. If there is excessive crying, a pacifier will sometimes help him settle, or simply changing his sleep position.

2. If your baby is habitually waking up 45 minutes into his nap,

screaming in pain and inconsolable, consider going in after 40 minutes and gently rocking him through the cycle so he does not become over-stimulated by his crying.

3. For the baby over three months, try using a pacifier immediately upon waking; or if he is fully awake, pick him up and comfort him as best you can. Sit, walk or rock him until he displays signs of tiredness, and then try putting him back down.

Crying

1. Typical signs of reflux are crying through feedings, not latching on, very small feedings and crying until exhausted. Feed a very young baby immediately upon waking. Avoid letting your reflux baby get into a full cry.

2. Whenever a baby is showing signs of stress during a feeding, stop, soothe and relax your baby, and then continue feeding.

3. Since reflux infants tend to be more comfortable in an upright position, they generally object to being laid down, especially on their backs. While the AAP recognizes that the back position may increase crying with a reflux baby, the organization generally recommends the back sleeping position because of SIDS statistics. You will need to discuss this matter with your pediatrician for what is best for your baby's situation.

4. Remember to take one day at a time, focusing on the long-term goal of establishing healthy feed/wake/sleep cycles. Some days will go well, and other days you will have to regard as stepping stones toward the big picture. All of parenting is a process, but especially with a reflux baby; so be patient with yourself and baby. It will probably take a few extra weeks before he stabilizes his routine, but he will get there.

WHATEVER HAPPENED TO THE BABIES?

From Ashley's journal: "Once Asher was diagnosed with reflux, we knew what we were up against and that made caring for the little guy that much easier. Asher improved greatly with the help of medication, and by six months his acid reflux problem was gone. It was then he began to sleep through the night. (He was night trained in three days.) Once he started sleeping through the night, he simultaneously developed a much better napping routine. He eventually moved to two naps a day, about 1½ hours each (morning and afternoon). Today, at two years of age, we constantly have people amazed at how well Asher goes to sleep at night. He still sleeps 12 hours and naps 2 to 3 hours."

From Stephanie's journal: "Because of his healthy weight gain, Caleb's pediatrician chose medication over any invasive procedures. The meds worked wonderfully. His reflux improved beautifully, and most significant of all, his little body began to relax. After a week of this, Caleb went to bed and slept 12 hours through the night, and he has continued to do so ever since."

From Whitney's journal: "At his three-month checkup, Micah was placed on Prevacid® and that fixed the problem. He transitioned to his crib and began sleeping through the night. At 15 months of age, we dropped the medication completely. His 18-month checkup was encouraging. For the first time, Micah was above the 50 percent range. In hindsight, I was discouraged by how many people told me, 'All you really have is a laundry problem.' Not true! The information I wished I had beforehand was the best way to continue working on a routine with a reflux infant without thinking he should be sleeping through the night at eight weeks. I learned reflux babies are delayed in this category, and that is not a reflection on either the baby, the parent or *Babywise*; it is just a normal outcome for a reflux baby."

From Sally's journal: "We took a list of symptoms to our pediatrician, who immediately suspected reflux. She prescribed

Zantac®. We saw a significant difference in Ross in two days. As he began feeding better, his day and night sleep also improved. Ross continued nursing for 13 months. Once he started drinking from a cup, we stopped the medicine. The reflux was gone."

SUMMARY

Caring for a baby with colic, reflux or GERD, is a major task that can be very stressful for the entire family. For that reason, parents should get medical help for their baby as quickly as possible. They will do better if they can humbly ask or receive help from family and friends who can provide meals and give them a needed break. Parents should not be afraid to let trustworthy people care for their baby, so they can rest. Caring for this little life can and should be a team effort.

For more information on nutrition, allergies, Lactose Intolerance, GERD and other health related matters, please connect with us at: *www.Facebook.com/BabywiseLife*.

Chapter Nine

Topic Pool

When a couple learns they have conceived, not much initially changes in their daily routine. Their domestic and professional duties continue as before with very little disruption. Mom will make some gradual adjustments as the baby grows within, but overall, life on the pre-birth side of things is much easier than after delivery. Then comes Baby! While the probability is very high that Mom will experience a normal pregnancy and birthing process, it is unlikely that once Baby comes home everything will go exactly as Mom and Dad envisioned. Like the New Year's resolutions people make in December, the *reality* of January has a way of throwing them off course. Newborns can do this to parents.

Expectations versus reality will always be part of parenting. What expectant couple does not, at least for a moment, believe things will be different for them than for the struggling couple down the street? Most women possess a quiet confidence that their pregnancy will be different, their ability to manage a newborn will be without challenge, their home life will quickly return to normal, and their baby will respond with sweet smiles and contented coos to every motherly gesture of love and care. While we have no desire to dampen anyone's enthusiasm or hopeful expectations, we offer this caution to help you: the more you leave room in your thinking that babyhood comes with a few unplanned disruptions, the better you will be able to adjust when the unexpected invades your baby's day. Parents who assume they can plan and control every moment without some sort of intrusive disruption will feel disappointed. By accepting the reality that they cannot, in a God-like fashion, control all outcomes of their baby's life, they are accepting their humanity. In time they will learn how to manage the unexpected. To help minimize the adjustments a new baby brings into your home, we now discuss an alphabetical listing of topics helpful to think through before your baby arrives. Some of the topics were mentioned in previous chapters, but warrant further discussion.

ACHIEVEMENT LEVELS

All human beings are uniquely different, yet we share developmental similarities that serve as a basis for achievement levels. A basic routine enhances learning because order and predictability are natural allies of the learning process. Keeping in mind the ripple-effect principle, good routines encourage healthy sleep, and good sleepers experience optimal alertness during waketimes. That facilitates how they interact with their environment. As a result, these children are self-assured and happy, less demanding and more sociable, secure and healthy. They have longer attention spans, possess self-control and focusing skills, and as a result, become faster learners.

There is uniformity within infant development, which means infants differ only slightly in the age at which they achieve new levels. If your baby seems to be at a slower pace than your neighbor's baby, that is not an automatic cause for concern. One baby cuts a tooth at four months and another baby at six months. That is not a problem, just a difference, reflected in the range of norms you will see in baby books (including this one).

If, however, your baby does not achieve a skill within the norm tables of expectations, that could signal a muscular or neurologic problem. For example, pediatricians are concerned when a full-term two-month-old is not able to lift his head while lying on his tummy. They are also concerned if a full-term three-month-old is crossing his legs when lifted under his arms, or if his neck lacks muscle control to support his head when picked up from a back-lying position. Understanding the various developmental markers of growth can help parents make a general assessment of their baby's progress. If you sense your baby is lagging behind developmentally, consult your healthcare provider. The term *developmental delay* is applied to infants who are not growing according to established norms.

Premature infants, who comprise about 12 percent of U.S. babies, have a different set of norms and will lag behind full-term infants in achievement levels up through the first two years. Happily, they usually catch up with full-term babies in every category of development by age two.

BABY EQUIPMENT

With the exception of the car seat and the crib, other baby equipment is optional. It is easy to walk into a baby super store and get caught up with the new, the pretty, and the fancy. Baby equipment and accessories are marketed to parents' likes and preferences. In truth, your baby doesn't care about fashion. It is simply not on their radar, so do not worry if new or pretty are not supported by your budget. Many items, including the high chair, stroller, changing table and crib can be borrowed from a relative or friend, or found at a garage sale. (For the latest product reviews, DIY ideas, and innovations, visit us at *www.babywise.life/babygear.*)

Baby Monitor

Audio baby monitors first came on the scene in the 1960s. Today's generation of monitors now include video capability. Parents can hear and see what is going on in baby's room. The price tags range from $30 for a simple monitor without video to $400 if you are looking for High Definition color and night vision.

Some kind of monitor is worth the investment, because it allows you to monitor your baby from a distance. This provides

Mom and Dad the extended freedom to move around the house while Baby is in his crib, playpen or eventually playing by himself in his room. A potential downside is that hearing every little sigh, noise, whimper or stirring a baby makes is cute at first but can become wearying. And in the still of the night, monitors magnify every sound, leaving parents in a state of exhaustion by morning. The last thing a baby needs in the morning is a cranky parent, so consider turning the sound control down at night. Be aware that baby monitors are not medical devices and are not intended or able to prevent SIDS.

Car Seat

The car seat is an item that will be around for a while, so think long-term when making this investment. Some car seats are very stylish and work fine with an infant but may not be practical for a growing toddler. To avoid having to purchase a second car seat, do some comparison shopping.

For first time parents it's important to understand the additional attention to be paid to protect your baby when he's traveling in his car seat. To prevent your baby's head from rolling side to side and potentially causing damage to his neck muscles, considering rolling a cloth diaper or receiving blanket to support each side of the baby's head. Or you can purchase special inserts made for car seats. Whatever you choose, be sure the items does not block your baby's breathing.

With precious cargo on board you will drive cautiously and defensively being mindful that sudden stops impact babies most of all because they lack neck-muscle strength. Infants and toddlers should ride in a rear-facing seat until they reach the weight or height designated for their car safety seat manufacturer. Most seats allow children to ride rear facing for at least two years.

Crib

Cribs and cradles are not products of the Industrial Revolution but pieces of furniture that have been around for thousands of years. Ancient Mediterranean societies from Greece, Rome and Israel all used cribs for their babies. The cradle, an infant crib with rocking motion, gained popularity in the Middle Ages and became a status symbol of wealth. Mothers in primitive settings hung cribs from the ceiling of their huts, where they could gently rock their babies as they passed by. The crib is the most basic piece of baby furniture you will own. Give thought to the one you will buy or borrow, since your child will spend nearly half of the first 18 months of his life in it.

A firm, good quality mattress should fit snugly against all four sides of the crib. A snug fit prevents the baby from getting any body parts stuck between the mattress and the crib. The guardrail should be at least 26 inches above the top of the mattress to discourage any attempt to climb out when the baby is older.

The spaces between the crib slats should be no more than 2 and 3/8 inches apart. A crib bumper guard is a good investment and safer for the baby than using pillows or stuffed animals, which could cause suffocation. Avoid placing the crib near drafty windows, heaters or air ducts. A steady blast of hot air can dry out your baby's nose and throat, leading to respiratory problems. The AAP does not recommend placing a baby to sleep on a soft surface such as a water bed, pillow or soft mattress.

Infant Seat

This is not a car seat. An infant seat is a lightweight, portable seat made especially for infants. You can use it from day one and will find it more useful than any other piece of equipment in the early weeks and months. Infant seats will often come with chair straps for safety sake, which makes it suitable for feeding your baby solids, when the time comes. While the highchair will be used most of the time, the infant seat is handy, especially when out visiting friends or at a restaurant.

Infant Swings

Some infant swings play music while they rock, and others offer a variety of reclining options and multiple speeds. Babies going through fussy times tend to soothe more quickly in a swing set at a fast pace, whereas a slower speed is conducive for relaxed, non-fussy times. The reclining swing also works well after feeding to help relieve pressure in Baby's full tummy.

The AAP recommends not using the swing until your baby is capable of sitting up on his own, usually by 7-8 months of age. Most grandmothers, however, will tell you that once your baby has good head and upper-back control, the swing can be introduced in the reclining position, as long as the baby is propped well and firmly secured so he cannot move or slip out of the swing.

A swing should not be used for long periods of time, no more than 15-20 minutes twice a day, and never out of Mom or Dad's visual range. When using the swing for Baby so that you can accomplish a task like preparing dinner, make a point of talking to your baby while he is swinging.

Whether you purchase a new swing or borrow one from a friend, make sure it is assembled well and has a wide base and low center of gravity. While tipping over is rare, it can happen if the swing is not centered correctly, and your baby leans too far over in one direction. Use the lap and shoulder belts faithfully—they are there to protect your baby!

Playpen

Once parents have their infant's feeding and sleeping routines under control, then it is time to work on Baby's waketime activities. Parents can begin using the playpen as a portable bed soon after their baby is born and for tummy time once the baby can hold his head up and is able to explore an item in his hands. Once your baby is able to sit up by himself, playpen time should become a routine part of his day. We explain in detail the developmental benefits of this in *Babywise II*.

BATHING YOUR BABY

Babies should not receive their first full bath until the umbilical cord has fallen off (10-14 days after birth on average). Never immerse your baby in water while the cord is still attached. A sponge bath is all a newborn really needs. Never try to remove the umbilical cord by cutting or twisting it off. It will fall off by itself any time after the second week of age. Keep the cord-area clean by using a cotton swab and some rubbing alcohol or by using alcohol wipes. This should be done after each diaper change.

After the cord falls off, and your baby is ready for a bath in the kitchen sink (easier on your back) or baby's bathtub, be sure the water is warm to the touch but never hot. Go easy on the soap since it is drying to the skin, leaving it itching and flaky.

Never leave a baby in water unattended, even after he is capable of sitting up by himself. The potential danger is too great a risk, even for a minute.

BLANKET TIME

It may be hard to imagine that learning could be taking place when a five-month-old baby is stretched out on his blanket, playing with a colorful toy or teething ring, yet it is true; blanket time facilitates early learning by allowing a baby to concentrate and serves as a useful mobile boundary. Begin blanket time with your baby as soon as he is able to hold his head up and manipulate an object in his hands, as early as four months. Start with 5-10 minutes once a day and stretch the time to a level contentedly accepted by your baby. The beauty of a blanket is its mobility. You can place it just about anywhere in the house convenient for Mom and Dad. Grandparents will also find it helpful when the baby is over for a visit.

BONDING WITH YOUR BABY

The term, "bonding," evolved from a controversial theory in

the 1980s relating to mothers and their babies into common usage today to describe two people emotionally connecting. The original theory postulated that a sensitive period exists for the mother soon after birth when she must make eye-to-eye and skin-to-skin contact with her baby for a long-term maternal connection to truly take place. Most couples assume this bonding is for the baby's benefit, but the theory focuses on the mom, suggesting that if she fails to make an immediate connection right after birth, she is more likely to reject her baby passively by withholding love and nurturing. Before worrying about the poor mom who does not have the chance to hold her baby immediately after delivery, be aware that *research has not substantiated* the cause-and-effect relationship this theory speaks of. Although some animals show instinctive tendencies of this sort, speculating that rational beings respond similarly is scientifically unacceptable. Anthropology, the study of humankind, is very different from zoology, the study of animals.[1]

The shortsightedness of the bonding theory, however, should not take away from the beautiful moment right after birth when Mom, Dad and Baby meet for the first time. There should be plenty of touch, tears, photos, and soft words of affection. If Mom and Baby are temporarily separated at birth, her love as a mother will not diminish, nor will her child move through life permanently impaired because of a bonding deficit created in the first few hours or even days after birth.[2]

CESAREAN BIRTH

This method of delivery, commonly referred to as a C-section, is accomplished through an incision in the abdominal wall and uterus. The decision to perform a C-section is made either prior to your due date because of a known condition or unexpected complication, or during labor because of an unexpected complication. In either case, competent doctors have your best interests in mind.

Often a first-time mom goes into labor before having a

C-section, which means her body must endure two major events, and so must Baby. Infants born by emergency C-sections tend to experience a bit more sluggishness or fussiness for the first few weeks. They may be cranky because of medications Mom must take post-op, but typically everything settles down by the third week. C-section babies experience no delays in sleeping through the night in the *PDF* population.

Because a Cesarean birth is major surgery, give yourself time to heal when you get home with the baby. When he naps, make sure you nap, too. Household chores can wait.

More C-sections are performed today because medical science has developed greater technology for protecting babies, but also because there are more lawsuits against obstetricians and gynecologists, forcing them to exercise conservative, lower-risk treatment. Having a C-section is a medical decision that in no way reflects on a woman's motherhood. The main goal of a C-section is a healthy outcome.

CRADLE CAP

As adults we shed skin cells frequently without noticing. With babies, the new skin cells grow rapidly and often faster than the old cells can fall off, leaving the old cells stuck to the new ones. When this happens, it appears as a white scaly or patchy rash. It tends to happen most often on a baby's head, ears and forehead and has acquired the name of cradle cap. It is not dangerous or contagious and bothers Mom and Dad more than Baby. Your healthcare provider will probably recommend a cream, along with the advice to monitor it, but not to worry about it.

CRIB DEATH (SIDS)

The unexpected death of a healthy baby is referred to as Sudden Infant Death Syndrome (SIDS) or crib death. It is responsible for about 7,000 reported deaths a year worldwide, and it is neither predictable nor preventable from what we currently know. There are more male victims, especially among those who are born prematurely, and it occurs more often among babies of certain ethnic groups, young single mothers, and homes with at least one smoker. A child can be a victim of SIDS any time during the first year but the highest percentage occurs between months two to four. More babies die of SIDS during the winter months and in colder climates.

The research strongly suggests that putting a baby on his back for sleep rather than on his tummy reduces the risk of SIDS.(3) What is not conclusive is whether sleeping on his back is the primary or secondary factor in the reduction of risk. Is the risk removed because the child is sleeping on his back, which keeps his mouth and nose from directly laying on soft surfaces and gas-trapping objects (mattresses, pillows, crib liners)? Could those items be the actual sources of SIDS or is the problem connected to the biomechanics of tummy sleeping? More research is needed to answer those questions. Meanwhile, we suggest you speak to your health-care provider if you have any questions about positioning your baby for sleep, and do not worry about back positioning interfering with the establishment of healthy sleep patterns. We have not found any indications that it does.

DIAPERS, HYGIENE AND RASHES

As new parents, you have a choice between disposable or cloth diapers. It really is a matter of personal preference. As a general rule, you will change your baby's diaper at each feeding. *PDF* babies average 6-8 diaper changes a day, coinciding with their feedings. An exception is after the middle-of-the-night feeding, unless it is soaked or soiled or accompanied by a diaper rash, since your goal is to help your baby sleep through the night. When your baby finally begins to make the long 8-10 hour stretch through the night, use a diaper size larger than what you are using during the day or use two cloth diapers.

Since the skin of a newborn is so sensitive, it is best to use water and a clean cloth. Should you choose to use commercial wipes be sure they are specifically designed for newborns. Whatever baby wipe you choose they should be mild and free from alcohol and perfume.

When cleaning your baby, always work from front to back (never back to front), especially on girls to prevent the spread of bacteria that can cause urinary-tract infections. Pay attention to the creases in the thighs and buttocks. For boys, a good practice to develop is holding a clean diaper over his genitals, because exposure to air often causes boys to urinate with no regard for who is in the line of fire!

Wherever there is a diaper, there' is always the potential for a diaper rash. The rash may be caused by a yeast infection, food allergies, teething or sitting too long in a messy diaper. If your baby has particularly sensitive skin, he may be more prone to diaper rash. The best way to prevent diaper rash is to keep your baby's skin as dry and clean as possible, which means changing diapers as often as needed, preventing urine and other excrement from irritating the skin.

With proper attention and over-the-counter creams, most diaper rashes vanish in a few days. If your baby is on any medication, check the labels for side effects. If a rash persists, visit your healthcare provider for professional diagnosis and treatment. Read more about diaper rash care and treatment in Appendix One.

FEVERS AND SICKNESS IN NEWBORNS

When your newborn shows signs of sickness or has a fever above 100.4 degrees, contact your pediatrician immediately. A fever in a young baby is of great concern to pediatricians. It can indicate a wide variety of infections—ear, bladder, kidney or lung, perhaps—that only a professional can pinpoint. Although a fever is a sign that your baby's immune system is fighting off an infection, please stay mindful that a baby's immune system is not fully engaged until three months, leaving newborns more vulnerable to infection. Sickness and fevers are a natural part of life, but fortunately we live in a time when most common bacterial and viral infections are easily treated with medical intervention.

GRANDPARENTS

There is a special relationship between the third generation and the first. Within reason, you will want to take advantage of every opportunity for grandparents to enjoy your child. However, do not assume your parents want to baby sit, and do not abuse their generous offers to do so. Above all else, do not surrender your parenting responsibilities to your parents. While they may enjoy their grandchildren very much and probably have a few good opinions about parenting, they are not the parents—you are. We suggest you provide grandparents with their own copy of *Babywise*, so they know what you are doing and why. That way your baby has a team on his side!

Here we wish to leave a message for Dad: Many grandparents travel a great distance when the Big Day arrives. Of course, there is excitement and great anticipation, but that visit can either be a blessing or a problem, depending on your relationship with them and how like-minded they are with you. You might request that they postpone their visit until a few days or a week after the baby comes. By then you will have worked through your basic parenting routine and feel familiar with it. Having a high-powered, take-charge relative come in right after birth is very hard on a new mother's emotions. Dad can help by protecting his wife from that kind of stress and managing the situation for everyone's benefit.

IMMUNIZATIONS

The ability to protect children from the tragedies of many infectious diseases such as Polio, Diphtheria, and Measles is one of the great blessings of our day. To bring this blessing into your home, make sure your children receive all their recommended immunizations, and that they receive them on time. Because immunization schedules change frequently as better vaccines become available, routinely ask your pediatrician for a current timetable of vaccinations for your child from now through college. The latest recommendations at this writing from the Center for Disease Control and Prevention for infants include:

Hepatitis B vaccine
Rotavirus vaccine
Diphtheria and tetanus toxoids and acellular pertussis vaccine (DPT)
Haemophilus influenza type b
Pneumococcal vaccine
Inactivated poliovirus vaccine
Influenza vaccine (seasonal)
Measles, mumps, and rubella vaccine (MMR)
Varicella (chickenpox) vaccine
Hepatitis A vaccine

While the Internet is a valuable resource for health information, many websites contain false and misleading information about the safety of vaccines. We are commonly asked about the controversy surrounding "Dr. Bob's" Alternative Vaccine Schedule and what experts, with good reason, call a complete "misrepresentation of vaccine science." Please see the public warnings and statements from the AAP, the ACP (American College of Pediatricians) and the CDC (Center for Disease Control and Prevention) in Atlanta.

Consult your baby's pediatrician if you have questions about vaccines and immunization in general, but please get your children vaccinated!

MICROWAVE AND THE BOTTLE

For babies receiving formula, Mom or Dad will naturally want to take advantage of the microwave to heat a bottle of formula. *Loosen the top of the bottle to allow for heat expansion so it does not literally explode*. Be aware that microwaves heat food unevenly, creating hot spots, so be sure to shake the bottle well after heating and squirt a dab of milk on your wrist to test for warmth.

Since excessive heat can destroy the nutrient quality of expressed breastmilk, we recommend that you avoid using the microwave to thaw or heat it. Instead, place the bottle of expressed breastmilk in a bowl or small pan of warm water.

Whether your baby is getting breastmilk or formula, most will take a bottle at one time or another. It is important to keep the bottles and nipples clean and sterilized. This is safest with a bottle sterilizer designed to work in your microwave. They are available at major stores that sell baby items and come in various models and price ranges. A dishwasher can do the job with cages that hold the nipples and other small items, but only if you tend to wipe your dishes and utensils visibly clean before loading them (that is, you do not treat your dishwasher like a garbage disposal). It helps to shake down the bottles and other items that retain water when the rinse cycle stops so they dry properly during your dishwasher's drying phase.

NURSING TWINS

The *Babywise Parent-Directed Feeding* philosophy is a good friend to parents of multiples, especially in giving helpful advice about breastfeeding. Our experienced moms of twins find it best to assign a breast to each baby, and to keep them nursing on that specified breast throughout all feedings. This will help your milk supply keep up with the unique demand of each twin. Let one twin set the pace, and keep them both on that schedule. If that means you must wake one, do so.

During the first few weeks post-partum, you can nurse your twins simultaneously using a football hold—arms bent to support the back and head of each baby while they nurse. As they grow, your babies will have to nurse one at a time. Beyond that distinction, you will be able to implement all other aspects of the *PDF* plan, including feeding routines and sleeping through the night. May you thoroughly enjoy your double portion! (Our next chapter discusses multiple births.)

PACIFIERS AND THUMB-SUCKING

There are many good reasons for using a pacifier with your newborn. It can help satisfy a baby's non-nutritive sucking need; it is soothing and can preempt periods of stress; and it is useful when Mom needs a few more minutes before she can get to the baby for a feeding. Furthermore, research suggests pacifiers may help reduce the risk of SIDS.

There are, however, a few warnings. *First, the pacifier should not be introduced too early if Mom is breastfeeding.* There is the possibility that Baby might prefer the pacifier over Mom because nursing requires more energy. Second, since the pacifier is a source of pleasure, *it can become addictive*. For example, a baby may depend on it to fall asleep or fall back to sleep if waking early from a nap. Early on the pacifier can be a parent's friend, but stay mindful that it does not, in six to eight months, become Mom and Dad's foe.

Children—infants, pretoddlers, and toddlers—suck thumbs and fingers out of habit more out of a than a deep-seated psychological need for comfort. Infants find thumb-sucking soothing during times of stress, fatigue or calm. Unlike the pacifier, the thumb is physically attached to the child and the child can become habitually attached to the thumb. The good news is that 50 percent of infants give up thumb-sucking on their own by six to seven months of age. If either thumb-sucking or the pacifier becomes a problem after this period, you will find solutions spelled out in *Babywise II*.

PREMATURE BIRTH

While the normal full term gestation period is 40 weeks, a baby born from 37 weeks on is still considered full term. Babies born prior to 37th completed weeks of pregnancy are considered premature. In the 1980s, the rate of premature births fell to 3-5 percent. Today that rate is approaching 13 percent. There are two explanations for this sharp rise: the number of multiple births has increased from advancements made with in-vitro fertilization, and the advances in obstetrics and neonatology have improved the chances of survival for even the smallest babies, even those born as early as 24 weeks after conception.

Today, thanks to medical science, babies born at 24 weeks have a 60 percent chance of survival. At 26 weeks, survival rates jump to 86 percent. Preemies that make it to 32 weeks have a 99 percent chance of survival and a very low risk of health and development complications.

While most premature babies are at risk for some health problems, the closer to full term the baby is born, the less risk there is for serious complications. Size is also an issue for the premature infant. A baby born at 32 weeks will be significantly smaller than a baby at 40 weeks. That causes feeding challenges because preemies are sluggish eaters and can only take in small amounts of food. Pediatricians who specialize in high-risk premature births usually recommend calorie and vitamin-enriched formulas or that fortifiers to be added to breastmilk.

Since premature births are not planned, being aware of the possibility and understanding the risks will help any parent cope with the unexpected. There are many reputable medical websites that provide up-to-date information and the opportunity to ask questions related to premature births.

POSTPARTUM DEPRESSION (PPD)

Until Baby is sleeping at least 6 hours or more during the night, Mothers usually fight some level of fatigue. However, if you find that after your six-week postpartum check-up you are experiencing strong mood swings, have difficulty accomplishing minimal household tasks, or are constantly on the verge of tears during the day, please talk to your obstetrician. This state of mind and level of emotions at this point is not normal and is a symptoms of postpartum depression (PPD). The phone call to your doctor is free but the cost to yourself and the rest of your family is more than you probably will want to pay emotionally if you do not get help.

There are three levels of postpartum hormonal imbalance. The first and least serious level, the *Baby Blues*, is something most women experience right after birth. It usually peaks around the forth or fifth day postpartum and typically disappears within ten days to two weeks. Moms experiencing the baby blues tend to cry over the smallest incidents, feel overwhelmed, lose their concentration easily and have some difficulty sleeping. Unlike postpartum depression, the baby blues is not an isolated condition. It can share the stage with Mom's feelings of joy, excitement and happiness.

The second level of hormonal imbalance is *Postpartum Depression* (PPD), which can set in a few days or even weeks after birth and considered by health-care authorities, to be a more serious condition than a simple case of baby blues. Mothers experiencing PPD have feelings of depression, sadness, hopelessness, despair and fatigue. They are often anxious, irritable, weepy, and unable to concentrate, and they can experience sleep and eating imbalances. A mother can greatly minimize the symptoms of PPD by keeping herself and her baby on a good routine, which allows her to get quality rest and proper nutrition. If she finds she is still abnormally melancholy after several weeks, she should pursue the counsel of her obstetrician.

The third level of imbalance linked to childbirth is *Postpartum Psychosis*. This is by far the most serious emotional state, since it usually causes a break from reality. Symptoms include hallucinations, delusions, suicidal or homicidal thoughts, and disorganized thinking. A mother who has been previously treated with a bipolar disorder is more likely to develop postpartum psychosis. Moms who suffer from this should see a physician as soon as possible. One in every 1,000 women who give birth suffers from this condition. This is no small matter, and the condition should be treated with a sense of urgency.

STARTING SOLID FOODS

Introducing solid foods into a baby's diet does not mean stopping liquid feedings. The calories gained from breastmilk or formula are still of prime importance, but now your baby has reached a growth point at which liquid feedings alone are no longer nutritionally sufficient.

Babies usually start solid food between four to six months. Although the AAP leans more toward six months, your pediatrician will direct you based on your baby's unique nutritional needs. There are developmental signs to look for before offering solids. Your baby must be able to control his neck and head muscles and sit upright (with support). This skill level usually aligns with the baby who can lift his head off a blanket and sustain that position longer than a minute.

Other indicators of readiness include your baby showing signs of hunger even thought he is receiving 32 ounces of formula a day. If breastfeeding, he is showing signs of hunger after 6-8 full feedings in a 24-hour period. The baby who has a well-established nighttime sleep pattern and then between 16-24 weeks begins to walk at night, or early during well established naps may also be signaling the he needs more nutrition. See *Babywise II* for specific details about adding solids to your baby's diet.

SWADDLING A BABY

Most newborns enjoy the security that comes from being swaddled. This age-old practice which we encourage helps to calm and comfort a fussy baby, facilitates sleep with a newborn and minimizes the startle reflex that can often wake a sleeping baby. Learning how to swaddle a baby is not difficult. Use a regular receiving blanket or a swaddle blanket.

We offer a few cautions: be careful not to swaddle the baby too tightly, since that restricts breathing and circulation, and be careful that the blanket does not cover the baby's face. There will come a time, of course, when your baby no longer enjoys being swaddled and will let you know. Just follow your baby's lead on this.

TEETHING

Teething is the term used when a tooth begins to break through the gum and is all part of normal growth. It usually starts between five to seven months. Generally the lower two teeth come in first followed by the upper, middle-two teeth. Teeth tend to erupt sooner in girls than boys, but around two years of age both boys and girls have, or are close to having, all 20 of their baby teeth.

Teething should not interfere with breastfeeding since the sucking reflex used while nursing is done by the tongue and palate, not the gums. Discomfort, irritability, fussiness, increased salivation and a slightly-raised temperature might accompany the eruption of a tooth but should not produce any change in your baby's feeding routine. You may find that teething causes a mild disruption with your baby's sleep but not enough to override a well-established sleep pattern.

Your child should see a dentist around the time his first tooth comes into his mouth; but at the very least, make sure your child sees a dentist for a well-baby dental check-up by his first birthday. This is very important because early evaluation and education are the keys to preventing childhood dental diseases. Your dentist can help you determine your child's risk for tooth decay and help you with techniques to clean his teeth effectively and safely. Starting to visit the dentist at an early age helps your child become comfortable in a dental office.

WEANING YOUR BABY

Weaning is the process by which parents offer food supplements in place of or in addition to mother's milk. That process begins the moment parents offer a bottle of formula, or when their baby first tastes cereal. From that moment on, weaning is a gradual process. As it relates to breastfeeding, there is no set age that weaning is best or preferable.

When ready, a breastfeeding mom can start the weaning process by eliminating one feeding at a time, going three to four days before dropping the next one. That time frame allows Mom's body to make the proper adjustments in milk reduction. Usually the late-afternoon feeding is the easiest one to drop since it is a busy time of day. Replace each feeding with 6-8 ounces of formula or milk, depending on the child's age. (Pediatricians generally recommend babies not receive whole milk (cow's milk) until they are at least one year old.) While Baby may not wean from the breast or bottle before his first birthday, Mom must think ahead by introducing the "sippy cup" around six to seven months of age. *Babywise II* covers the practical side of this feeding option.

For the formula-fed baby, moms can begin making the transition from the bottle to the sippy cup around 10-11 months of age. When you begin to wean from the bottle, start with the Noon meal. A few days later, eliminate the morning and late-afternoon bottles. The evening bottle will be the last to go. This process takes time, so be prepared and be patient.

With additional articles, books, research, and *Babywise* Mom feedback we are constantly updating our *www.Facebook.com/BabywiseLife*. resource center. This is a good place to connect with other *Babywise* Moms. For more helpful tools and tips, sign up for our newsletter.

Chapter 10

Multiple Births

The Endless Party

by Eleanor Womack, M.D.

A baby is a great blessing, and multiple births represent multiplied blessings to parents. However, with twins, triplets or more, your joy will be accompanied by a great deal of work. This is a matter of simple addition—no, make that multiplication!

All parenting requires organization and thinking ahead, but that is especially true with multiple births; because when the unexpected happens, it happens in multiples. People with a single baby make their mistakes one at a time; parents of triplets tend to make their mistakes in triplicate. On the bright side, when you do things right, you have multiplied success.

At our house we like to think of parenting our triplets as the party that never ends. When our three boys were tiny preemies and needed feeding every 3 hours, we saw feeding times as an opportunity for family fun and fellowship. The "feeders" would sit together in the same room and discuss their days, tell jokes or stories, or sing songs. Even at 3:00 a.m., we feeders were encouraged in our toil by our mutual commitment to see this as an opportunity to socialize.

From the earliest age, children sense your attitude. If you approach their care as a burden or drudgery, your children will respond in a burdensome way, and you will experience drudgery. Instead, see each day as an adventure and know that each stage of your children's development is precious.

BRINGING THEM HOME

Multiple-birth pregnancies are at high risk for prematurity. Therefore, a major challenge early on is caring for tiny babies in multiple. Your babies may stay in the hospital Neonatal Intensive Care Unit (NICU) for a while. They may come home one at a time as they reach safe weights and develop sucking skills. They may come home with apnea and heart monitors in tow. (The apnea monitor provides assurance a child is breathing.)

<u>Cribs</u>: When your babies are very young, they will not be moving around much on their own. It is perfectly acceptable to put two or even three small babies in the same crib. We suggest you separate them when they are mature enough to wiggle around in the crib, preventing any baby from becoming a suffocation risk to another.

<u>Diapers</u>: Triplets will use between 24-30 diapers a day, so the cost of diapers can become a significant item on the household budget. Weigh your options. For lowest cost up front, you may want to buy cloth diapers and wash them yourself. But when you factor in the need for daily loads of laundry, the cost in terms of time and inconvenience is considerable. Also, cloth has a hidden cost built in because of increased incidence of diaper rash. Babies cannot go as long between diaper changes in cloth as they can in disposable diapers because of the lower absorbency of cloth diapers and higher discomfort level when wet. Parents of multiples find it hard enough to keep track of who has been changed and who is due for a fresh diaper, let alone be aware of who is wet or dirty at an unexpected time.

Disposable diapers are helpful because babies do not experience discomfort even when a wet diaper is overlooked.

Commercial diaper services are cheaper than disposable diapers, but you will have multiple quantities of wet, smelly diapers waiting for pickup each week. I prefer disposable diapers, but because of cost concerns, I encourage parents to try a diaper service and see if they can keep the babies changed and comfortable. If this service works for you, you may realize significant savings.

YOU NEED HELP

As I counsel expectant mothers of multiples, the single worst mistake I see them make is assuming they can handle this challenge on their own. Frequently their budget is small and hired help is out of the question, so Mom and Dad set out to accomplish all childcare duties on their own. Do not make this mistake! You cannot do it alone.

You do not necessarily have to spend money to get help. There are several alternatives. Extended family members often love to help out, especially if your babies are eating and sleeping on a schedule. Some high schools, colleges, seminaries and yeshivas near your home may offer classes in childhood development. Your home could become a learning lab for some kindhearted students and their teacher. Churches and synagogues are filled with people available to lend a helping hand—you need only ask. If one or more of your children comes home using monitors, you may be a candidate for in-home nursing care, possibly at the state's expense. To find out about this possibility, check with the social worker associated with the neonatal intensive care unit of your hospital or your pediatrician.

When people ask if they can help, always say "Yes, please!" Keep a daily planner handy so you can give to all who offer help an exact date and time they can serve you—right there on the spot—and immediately assign them a job. You may want help with baby care, or if your volunteers have limited time, ask them to help with a predictable weekly task, such as the laundry and trips to the grocery store and pharmacy. Delegating is one of the keys to preserving your sanity with multiples

FEEDING MULTIPLES

Are you going to breastfeed? A mother of multiples often can breastfeed. Whether this is the right choice for you and your babies is up to you and your children to determine. Much will depend on your babies' maturity at birth and whether they require NICU care, whether you had a Cesarean section, and how many babies you have. Mothers of twins are more successful at breastfeeding than mothers of triplets. If your babies come right home with you from the hospital, it will be much easier to establish a breastfeeding pattern.

As explained in Chapter Four, mother's milk is a complete and perfect food. It is easily digested, provides excellent nutrition, and contains the right balance of proteins and fats. It also provides additional antibodies that help establish your baby's early immune system. If your babies are in the NICU, even if you do not plan to breastfeed them directly, you may want to provide milk for them using an electric breast pump. Many pediatricians recommend this, and insurance companies will often reimburse a mother for the pump rental while the baby is in the NICU. Premature babies especially will benefit from the antibodies in breastmilk, but do not feel guilty if providing mother's milk just does not work for you and assume your formula-fed babies will grow up sickly. It simply is not true.

Each of your babies is different. You may plan to breastfeed all of them but find that one prefers the bottle to the breast. Some moms successfully breastfeed all their multiples in a rotating fashion, with one baby receiving a bottle each feeding while the others have a turn at the breast. Other mothers produce enough milk to feed all three of their triplets. A good electric pump is very helpful in establishing and maintaining a milk supply for multiples. You may be able to pump after you feed one or two babies so that a third or fourth baby can receive breastmilk in a bottle. Breastfeeding can be magnificently easy once established and learned by Mom and babies, but it does not start out easy, especially after the stress of a high-risk pregnancy. Please relax your expectations of yourself and get good counsel from a professional lactation consultant. Breastfeeding multiple babies may not come naturally, and you probably will need guidance.

If your newborns have low birth weight and are premature, they will probably sleep almost all the time. You may find they hardly ever wake up, sleeping even when you are changing their diapers, bathing them, and feeding them. Premature babies react to stimulus by withdrawing and sleeping. Do not fight their sleepiness. Do your best to get the food into them but do not try for more than 30 minutes every 2½ to 3 hours. From the beginning of one feeding to the beginning of the next, no more than 3 hours should elapse. Attempt to feed and burp each infant for 30 minutes, putting the sleeping baby back to bed for the remaining 2 to 2½ hours of the cycle. Do this even if the baby was sucking ineffectively and only received a fraction of the usual feeding amount or when a significant amount of the feeding is spit back up. I recommend that you do not re-feed after a baby spits up if the 30-minute limit is up. If the baby spits up 10 minutes or so into the feeding, try re-feeding until the time is up.

One important aspect of feeding newborn and premature infants is a good assessment of their hydration. Each baby should have between 6-8 wet diapers each day. If you are breastfeeding, this will be one clue to help you determine that they are properly latched on and consuming adequate quantities of milk. But with a multiple birth, especially three or more babies, keeping track of who has or has not had a wet diaper can become a challenge. In the early sleep-deprived postpartum weeks, you can lose track of even obvious things; so write it all down. Keep your Healthy Baby Growth charts near the changing table and keep them updated. Try color-coding them, assigning a different color to each child. This will make it easier to keep track of each child's progress.

As your babies mature, feedings will become easier and you will probably be able to feed each baby in under 30 minutes. Adhere closely to the feeding /waketime/naptime order for each baby. When one wakes at night to eat, wake them all and feed them. However, when one wakes up early from a nap, resist the temptation to reward the baby with a feeding. Instead, check for a dirty diaper, calm the baby and lead the child into comforting himself and going back to sleep.

SLEEP FOR MULTIPLES

Sleep for multiples is crucial to their happiness and your peace of mind. With newborns—especially two or more small, premature babies—the temptation is to focus on how much they eat, how often they eat and whether they are gaining weight consistently. My husband and I have applied the *PDF* principles from birth with our triplets, and we have counseled many parents of multiples to do the same. The true key to eating and weight gain is sleep. If you want your children to eat and to grow, teach them to sleep. A rested baby will eat. An exhausted, agitated, sleep-deprived baby will howl, fuss, suck ineffectively and spit up repeatedly.

You may be afraid your babies will wake up hungry an hour after you put them down if they have not taken a full feeding. I was! The surprise is that they tend to wake up just in time for the next scheduled feeding, better rested and ready to take in a full meal. Overall, the newborn babies whose parents focus on sleep rather than calories will get more nutrition because they will be better rested, have better digestion, and be ready to suck strongly.

As your multiples mature, they will develop definite waketimes and sleep times. When they are newborn or premature, they will almost always fall asleep while you are feeding them, or maybe they will not even wake up for the feeding. As they get older, they will still get drowsy with feedings, but with a little stimulation, you can have them fully awake and ready to play after a meal. Waketime activities with multiples should always include some independent playtime. When the appointed time for the nap arrives, the babies may indicate readiness by being fussy and non-distractible, or they may be wide awake and cheery. Put them down awake! Logistically, you cannot rock two, three or more babies to sleep at each naptime. Your babies need to learn to comfort themselves. In fact, all babies need to learn patience and how to calm themselves as vital life skills. That Mom and Dad each have only one lap and one set of arms presents unavoidable limits. Self-comforting is particularly important when babies are sick or under stress. If they have learned the skill of sleep early on in life, they will seek sleep when they feel tired instead of further stressing themselves with crying and fussing.

If your multiple babies have been sharing a room since birth, they will not wake each other up. They will learn to shut out each other's crying, so do not separate them when one is fussing. When little ones are having a particularly hard cry, you can go in every 10 minutes to pat them, reassure them and possibly check for a wet or soiled diaper. You will function as a guide, teaching them how to self-comfort. Go in long enough to help them stop crying but not so long that they fall asleep. Your goal is to put them down awake, allowing them to fall asleep on their own—without a transition process, such as rocking or patting. This is more challenging than it sounds because of the sheer physical effort required to care for multiples.

You need to start and finish each feed-wake-sleep cycle in a fairly structured fashion. It takes about 15-20 minutes to pick up three babies, diaper them and put them in their cribs for a nap. One common pitfall for parents is to allow their babies to fall asleep in their waketime activity chairs or swings. Parents get busy doing a household chore, answering the phone or trying to solve one baby's problem, only to find the others have fallen asleep sitting up. While it is true they have fallen asleep by themselves, they did not do that in the right place—their own cribs. If that happens often, they may have difficulty learning to comfort themselves as they lie in their cribs. There will always be unexpected events to contend with, but try to plan ahead by putting your babies down awake in their cribs when you are not distracted. That way, when they fall asleep sitting up, it will be a rare event and not a habit.

Regarding sleep, the Number One question I receive from parents of multiples is this: "Our babies are about four months old and feeding every 4 hours but not sleeping through the night. Why?" I encourage those parents to try a rigorous 3-hour feeding schedule during the day and promote sleep at night. Usually, I get a call three days later to report the "miracle" that one or all the babies are now sleeping 8 hours at night!

Here is the first rule of nighttime sleep: Do not be tempted to lengthen the time between daytime feedings until your babies are sleeping at least 9 to 10 hours at night. They need the 3-hour feeding during the day to distinguish night from day but also to make sure their nutritional needs are being met. A basic 3-hour routine will accomplish both.

As they continue to mature, a brand-new issue arises: between six to nine months of age, your babies discover each other. That is when the party really begins! The nice problem you face is they are having too much fun entertaining each other. They will not wake up to each other's crying but will wake up to each other's laughter and carrying on. They have built-in buddies. What helps in this situation is for the early riser to have a toy to play with quietly in bed, while the siblings continue to sleep. In our family we place small, noiseless toys in each child's bed after the children have fallen asleep, so the one who wakes can play quietly and independently with the toy.

Strongly discourage your multiples from getting out of their cribs on their own. All babies should stay in their cribs until given permission, but for multiples there is an additional safety issue: the threat one aggressive toddler poses to another when unsupervised. We convinced our triplets that climbing in and out of their cribs was impossible without the help of a stepladder. When the stepladder was not available, they did not get in and out of their cribs. They slept in their cribs until after their third birthday without any episodes of unauthorized entry or exit.

ROUTINE FOR MULTIPLES

The routine of each baby should not vary, but the eat/sleep schedule of your multiple-birth babies with respect to one another may be affected by many factors. How many babies are there? How many feeders are there? Are you breastfeeding? Each baby should have feeding time, waketime, and naptime. Do not change that order, except for late-night feedings (when there is no waketime) and for premature babies who are not neurologically mature enough to tolerate waketime.

If you have triplets and there is only one caregiver for them most of the time, you may choose to stagger your babies' schedules. Here is how this might work. The feeder (probably you) starts the process on the hour with Baby A, finishes half an hour later and goes on to Baby B, while Baby A has waketime in a bouncy seat nearby. At the top of the next hour, Baby C wakes for feeding and Baby A is ready for naptime. When all three babies are fed, there are 1½ hours before the cycle starts again. If there are two feeders in your home, you could always have two babies eating at the same time.

With more help, all babies in a home with triplets or twins can be on approximately the same schedule. With two helpers, three babies can eat at the same time. Because babies eat at different speeds, there will be a fast eater and a slow eater. Once you figure out who eats slowest and who fastest, you can establish a system whereby one helper feeds the slow eater while the second helper feeds the fastest eater and the in-between eater. A breastfeeding mom can feed two babies at the same time while someone gives a bottle to the third baby.

WAKETIME

You will not need to focus on waketime during the first weeks your babies are home, but soon they will stay awake for the whole feeding and begin to take an interest in the world around them. A reclining upright seat is the perfect place to put a baby for these early waketime periods. The seat allows the baby to look around and wave his arms and legs while still upright, while at the same time discouraging him from spitting up, a common occurrence in babies who are lying horizontally. Reclining seats are useful later for feeding with a propped-up bottle or beginning solids when the babies are still too small for high chairs. Never leave a baby unattended in a seat, however.

Waketime activities for multiples do not require that you have three of everything. Babies tire of most activities after 10-20 minutes, so you can set up rotating play stations: one baby in a wind-up swing, another in a playpen with a rattle, and the third in a bouncy seat playing with a different rattle, or sitting with Mommy singing a song and playing one-on-one. At 15-minute intervals, rotate the babies to the next activity.

Individual time is essential to happy multiples. They need independent playtime each day, and they also need individual, one-on-one time with Mom and Dad. By necessity we tend to think of multiples as a unit. We feed, change, dress and bathe them all at the same time. It is much easier to make sure you are being fair and that everyone's needs are being met if you keep the babies on a schedule and do all major daily activities collectively. Nevertheless, how you structure waketime and the way you plan the babies' play activities can offer a break from the monotony of cookie-cutter baby care. For example, leave all but one of the babies with your spouse or a helper and take just one for a walk or on an errand to the store. Or read just one a story while the others play independently.

As multiples enter toddlerhood, they find themselves in a world where there is always someone else their size grabbing at them or at the toy they are about to pick up. Time in a playpen for a multiple becomes a time of refuge. They can do whatever they want in a playpen without someone interrupting them and taking their things. You can have one of nearly every other piece of equipment, but multiple playpens—one for each child—is a good early investment. Playpen time also provides a welcome relief for Mommy: she can answer the phone or make lunch while the children play safely. Begin to practice playpen time at three to four months of age. Start with just 10 minutes a day and slowly increase the time so that by one year of age, they can stay in the playpen for at least 40 minutes.

A WORD TO HUSBANDS

The key to harmonious family life is a healthy husband-wife relationship. All other relationships in the home are impacted—positively or negatively—by that primary family relationship. Work at it and guard it with your life! You will only be as good a parent as you are a spouse. That is why it is essential for Dad to help at home, especially with multiples. Your wife will be able to listen to, share, and enjoy you only if she feels your support and encouragement. Your wife is the chief feeder, diaper-changer, bather and teacher/entertainer of the set of babies entrusted to you. She has no down time: 24 hours a day she has to be calm and controlled, so she can make the important assessments and decisions that are part of your babies' daily life. The more you cherish and serve your wife, the more you will get back in the beautiful forms of a composed, wise mom and peaceful, secure children.

Explore *www.Facebook.com/Babywise.Life* for more resources for families with multiples, including more help for Dad's changing role and influence. Connect with other moms just like you.

Appendix One

Taking Care of Baby and Mom

The days and weeks soon after birth are a busy time for Mom and Dad, since the learning curve is steep in adjusting to a new baby at home. They have a heightened awareness to make sure everything is going according to what books and charts point to as normal, but the challenge for most first-time parents is discovering what "normal" looks like. We trust this section will help bring clarity to the issues that arise during these early weeks of adjustment.

This Appendix is divided into two sections: the newborn's development and growth characteristics that health care professionals will be looking for, and the physical and emotional challenges a mother might face postpartum. The more expectant parents understand the changes that will be taking place after the baby arrives, the better prepared they will be when even the unexpected happens.

Apgar Score

You have probably heard other parents talk about their baby's Apgar Score, but you may not have fully understood what it meant or how it is used to assess a newborn's health. The test was designed and perfected in 1952 by Dr. Virginia Apgar, who used it to determine the effects birthing anesthesia had on newborns. Eventually her test became the normative tool to help doctors determine the health status of babies at birth. The test measures five critical areas of newborn vitality within the first minute after birth and then five minutes later. Each point is given a value, and the sum total provides the score. A score of 7-10 is considered normal and indicates a baby in good condition. A score of 4-6 indicates a baby who probably needs respiratory assistance, and a score of 0-3 indicates the need for lifesaving intervention. Here is a basic Apgar Scoring Chart.

APGAR	0	1	2
Appearance *(Color)*	Blue or pale pink	Body pink, extremities blue	Pink
Pulse *(Heart Rate)*	Absent	Below 100/min	Above 100/min
Grimace *(Response to Stimulation)*	No response	Grimace	Lusty cry
Activity *(Muscle Tone)*	Absent	Some movement	Good movement
Respiration *(Breathing Rate)*	Absent	Slow, irregular, weak cry	Good, strong cry

NEWBORN BASICS

All newborns are endowed with similar needs, characteristics and reflexes that are considered normal and are all part of what makes us human. Discovering the uniqueness of your baby is more than a pastime; it is a necessity of true nurturing and begins with becoming familiar with a baby's physical characteristics. What do you need to know?

Characteristics of a Newborn

Head:

- Measures 25 percent of the baby's body size.
- Average circumference is 13-14 inches.

- Neck muscles are weak, so Baby's head needs support at all times.

Fontanels:

- Areas of the skull (soft spots) that are not yet joined but are held together by membrane tissue. (The soft spot is where the skull is not fully formed, allowing room for the brain's tremendous growth during the first year, when over 50 percent of your baby's total head growth occurs.)
- Anterior fontanel (on top of the head)—closes at approximately 18 months of age.
- Posterior fontanel (at the back of the head)—closes at approximately three months of age.

Hair:

- Some babies are born with a full head of hair; others have no hair at all.
- It is not uncommon for babies to lose some or all of their hair within weeks after birth.

Milia:

- Little white bumps resembling pimples on the baby's forehead, nose, and cheeks.
- Nearly 50 percent of newborns have the condition of Milia. It is not contagious, and most cases disappear within the first month of life; although in rare cases it could last up to three months. There is no treatment for this condition, except time.
- Exact cause is not known, but Milia may develop when tiny skin flakes become trapped in small pockets near the surface of the skin. Do not attempt to remove. Contact baby's doctor.

Eyes:

- Color: Caucasian babies are usually born with blue eyes

with their permanent eye color becoming evident between six months to one year of age. Babies of African and Asian descent are usually born with brown eyes and the color does not change.

- Newborns are born cross-eyed because of immature eye muscles. If your baby's eyes continue to wander after three months of age, contact your pediatrician.
- By six months, a baby's eyes should be focusing together. If they are not, ask your baby's pediatrician to refer you to an ophthalmologist.
- There may be swelling or discharge from your baby's eyes because of the antibiotics applied at birth.
- The tear ducts begin to produce tears around the second or third week of life.

Sensory: Vision

- Newborns possess full visual capacity in terms of eye mechanics, but the brain center controlling vision is not yet fully developed. This is why babies are born nearsighted, meaning objects far away appear blurry. It is estimated that infants are able to see objects about 8-14 inches away.
- At birth, babies see bright and contrasting colors. Their full color vision is not developed until approximately three or four months of age, when they can determine hues and light shades.

Sensory: Hearing

- A baby can hear fairly well, but not perfectly, right after birth. A Newborn Infant Hearing Screening Test is common practice and usually performed prior to a baby's hospital discharge. Ask your pediatrician if it is part of his or her discharge protocol.
- Infants tend to regard loud noises as disturbing and soft sounds as soothing.

Sensory: Taste and Smell

- Both are well-developed at birth.
- Researchers have found that many babies are able to differentiate between their mother's milk and the milk from another woman.

Skin:

- "Lanugo" or fine downy hair is sometimes present on a baby's body at birth. This is seen more frequently in premature infants and normally disappears within a few days or weeks on its own.
- Dry, scaly skin. Is sometimes associated with peeling and is seen two-three weeks following delivery, and in babies born after 40 weeks of gestation.
- Ruddy Skin. The newborn's skin often has a ruddy hue, and for the first few days the hands and feet can have a bluish tint. As the baby's circulation improves, his skin color will become more consistent.
- Rash. A rash may develop if the baby is overdressed or wearing clothing made of an irritating fabric. About half of all newborns display a harmless rash of little red bumps that disappear on their own, usually within a week. If you have any concerns, contact your baby's healthcare provider.
- Birthmarks. There are a variety of classifications of birthmarks (such as "strawberry," port-wine stains and salmon patches) and moles that may appear at birth on newborns.
- "Mongolian spots." This is a purplish/bluish discoloration of the skin on the lower back or buttocks and normally disappears after the first year. These spots have no known anthropological connection to the people of Mongolia other than being more common in darker-skinned infants. At least one Mongolian spot is present on the majority of babies of Native American, African, Asian or Hispanic descent. Ten percent of Caucasian babies are born with such birthmarks.

Breathing:

- Newborn breathing rate: 30-60 breaths per minute. It is normal for breathing to be irregular and shallow. Some babies may be noisy breathers at night.
- Hiccups are normal, and many mothers know when their baby is having a bout during pregnancy. When the baby's diaphragm matures, the frequent hiccups disappear.

Extremities:

- A baby's arms and legs are disproportionately short for his body. It is also normal for the arms to be bent and held close to the chest with his little hands in a fist.
- Baby's legs are positioned similarly to that assumed in utero, and it is normal for most newborns to appear bow-legged.
- Nails are usually long at birth, soft and pliable. It is important to trim them weekly to prevent the baby from scratching his face. As babies grow and become more alert and aware of their surroundings, nail trimming becomes more of a challenge. The safest and easiest way to trim a baby's nails is when he is sleeping or right after his bath, when he is relaxed and his nails are slightly softer. Newborn baby clippers are available at your local drug store. (Do not use adult clippers on your baby.)

Reflexes:

- Certain reflexes are present at birth, most of which are vital for survival. They are also strong indicators of the vitality and health of the central nervous system and are often tested at the various well-baby checks. As the baby matures, it is normal for some reflexes to disappear and others to change. It is important for parents to have a basic understanding of how reflexes work, because they indicate how well their baby is doing and help pediatricians evaluate normal brain and neurologic activity. While there are about 90 named reflexes, here are the 10 most common: Sucking, Swallowing, Rooting, Gagging, Coughing, Grasping, Stepping, "Babinski," "Tonic Neck," and "Moro reflexes."

Sucking reflex

- This reflex was active in the womb and is very strong at birth, since it is required for feeding. Usually any stimulation of the baby's lips will elicit a sucking response. Babies often suck on their thumbs, fingers, or fists.

Swallowing reflex

- This reflex is also present before birth, as babies will swallow and then excrete amniotic fluid in utero.

Gagging reflex

- Prevents choking.

Rooting reflex

- This is when your baby turns his head in response to stimuli to receive food.

Coughing reflex

- This helps clear the air passages of mucus.

Grasping reflex

- If you place your finger inside the palm of your baby's hand, he will grasp it—often with enough strength to allow the baby's upper body to rise up.

Stepping reflex

- If the baby is held up under the arms in a standing position, his little legs will make walking motions.

Babinski reflex

- Many years ago, Dr. Joseph Babinski discovered that when he firmly stroke the sole of a baby's foot, the big toe turns up and the toes fan out. This reflex may continue up to two years of age. (If it continues after that, it may be a sign of some nerve damage.)

Tonic Neck reflex

- o This reflex, also called the Fencing reflex, happens when your baby turns his head to one side: his leg and arm on the same side will extend, while the opposite limbs bend. It is connected to your baby's ability to crawl on his hands and knees, which has other neurologic implications, and is one of the reasons Tummy Time for a young baby is so important.

Moro reflex

- o This happens when your baby is startled: his arms thrust out as if to embrace you and his legs straighten and stiffen. The Moro reflex is present in all newborns and usually remains until four to five months of age. Its absence at birth can indicate a problem.

CARING FOR YOUR NEWBORN

The following are routine baby-care practices that will become part of Mom and Dad's day.

Umbilical Cord Care

Shortly after birth, the umbilical cord is clamped and cut, leaving an inch-or-so stump that is saturated with a drying agent. Over the next several days the stump will turn black, and it usually falls off between the first or second week of life. Here are guidelines for umbilical cord care.

- Necessary equipment: cotton balls or swabs and rubbing alcohol. Saturate a cotton ball with rubbing alcohol and squeeze it over the stump. Take a cotton swab dipped in alcohol to wipe around the base of the stump. Follow this procedure at each diaper change to help dry the stump and prevent infection. To prevent the diaper from covering the stump, fold the front flap of the diaper away from Baby's stomach so the stump remains exposed.

- There normally is an unpleasant odor associated with the drying of the stump, but an excessively foul odor may indicate an infection. If you notice this problem, contact your healthcare provider.
- Call your pediatrician if there is excessive bleeding from the cord stump, pus-like drainage, or redness and swelling around the cord junction site.
- Until the cord stump falls off, avoid clothing that is binding around the waist.
- Do not immerse your baby in water for a bath until the stump has fallen off.
- Never attempt to remove the stump. It must fall off naturally.

Diapering

Diapering may seem intimidating the first few days, but it is a skill soon mastered. Parents can choose between cloth and disposable diapers. Read more about this in Chapter Nine.

When Your Baby Develops a Diaper Rash

- Most rashes occur because a baby's skin is sensitive and becomes irritated by a wet or messy diaper. If your baby has a diaper rash, change wet diapers frequently and as soon as possible after bowel movements.
- Clean the affected diaper area with warm water only (no wipes on a newborn, but you can use them later).
- Over-the-counter creams or powders specifically prepared for this purpose and applied on dry skin will usually clear up a mild rash.
- If a rash is present, leave your baby un-diapered and exposed to air for 30-minute periods, when possible.

If your is baby receiving antibiotics, you may notice a diaper rash suddenly appearing. That does not mean your baby is allergic to the antibiotic; rather it probably is a natural response to the change in the content and pH of his stool, which causes irritation to the skin. Do not stop the antibiotic unless advised by the pediatrician to do so.

Call the pediatrician if:

- o The rash continues or worsens for three days or longer.
- o The skin is bleeding or has blistered areas.
- o The area of the rash is swollen.

In these situations, over-the-counter creams and ointments will not help. Prescription medications will probably be necessary.

Bathing

During the first couple of weeks stay mindful not to immerse Baby in a sink or tub until the cord stump has fallen off, usually between 10-14 days. Until then, sponge bathing is all that is needed. Here are some guidelines to follow.

Bathing Guidelines:

- Gather everything needed before starting the bath.
- Ideally, bathe the baby during the warmest part of the day, keeping the room warm during the bath as well.
- When sponge bathing, keep baby covered with a blanket or towel except for the area being cleaned. Dry the baby immediately, as newborns lose body heat very quickly when wet.
- A baby tub that fits on a counter top or inside a regular tub is recommended, as it provides Mom or Dad greater control over the baby's body.
- Bath water should be comfortably warm, not hot.
- Until a baby can safely sit up (usually around six months

of age), he will need support while in the tub. Use your arm to support the baby's back while your hand holds his arm that is furthest away. This will provide you the greatest freedom, security and safety to wash your baby.

Circumcision Care

Circumcision is almost as old as history itself. The practice was historically (though not exclusively) a Jewish rite. Today, medical experts and studies affirm that there are modest benefits to circumcision, although not all agree on the necessity of it. Evidence suggests that circumcision may decrease the risk of urinary tract infection and that it virtually eliminates the possibility of cancer of the penis. Circumcision for infants is not a traumatizing experience; it is a minor surgery. The discomfort felt will be no more rooted in his memory than being pricked in the heel during his PKU blood test (a *phenylketonuria* test, which verifies that your newborn baby has an important enzyme). A circumcision normally heals within four to seven days and needs routine cleaning during diaper changes:

- Clean with a soft cloth and water; do not rub
- Apply a coat of Vaseline over the area of exposed tissue and cover with a gauze square. This protects the area from wetness and bacteria.
- Replace at each diaper change until area is healed.
- Call the pediatrician if there is excessive bleeding from the surgical site or if there is excessive swelling, redness, the presence of pus or drainage, or a foul odor.

JAUNDICE IN NEWBORNS

Jaundice is not a disease but a temporary condition characterized by a yellow tinge to the skin and eyes. The yellow comes from bilirubin (a bile pigment) in the blood and is usually easily controlled. If the condition appears more pronounced after the second day, frequent blood tests are taken and conservative treatment initiated.

Babies with moderately raised levels of bilirubin are sometimes treated with special fluorescent lights that help break down the yellow pigment. Additional fluid intake may also be part of the recommended treatment. In this case, your pediatrician may recommend other liquid supplements, although exclusive breastfeeding is usually the best way to correct this condition, even feeding as often as every 2 hours. Because bilirubin is eliminated in the stool, make sure your baby is having regular stools. A newborn with jaundice will tend to be sleepier than normal, so be sure to wake him for a feeding at least every 2½ to 3 hours.

SICK BABY CARE

While a sick baby can foster insecurity in the parents, they gain a new appreciation for the medical professionals that serve their baby during this time. It is normal for a baby to be sick as many as seven to nine times within the first year. Prevention is the best care so do what you can to provide your baby with a clean, safe environment and a routine that provides regular sleep, play, and feeding. If you observe any of the following symptoms, however, call your pediatrician:

- Rectal temperature over 100.4° F.
- Excessive vomiting or green vomit.
- Diarrhea, defined as three or more stools (watery or foul smelling) beyond what is normal for the baby and that continues for more than 48 hours.
- Constipation, defined as stools that are hard and dry or no stools for 48 hours. Remember that breastfed babies over a month old may have only one to two stools per week because breastmilk is nearly 100% digested. This is why it is important to know what is normal for your baby.

- Yellowish coloring of the skin and the whites of the baby's eyes.
- Baby is showing symptoms of dehydration. Similar to adults, babies become dehydrated when they do not receive enough liquids, but unlike adults, they cannot ask for or get a drink by themselves. In the first few weeks, babies may show signs of dehydration due to a breastfeeding problem. The warning signs include:
    - Lack of wet or dirty diapers
    - Dry tongue and mouth
    - Lethargic or difficult to wake for feedings
    - Weak suck or latching-on problems
    - Feeding less than eight times in 24 hours
    - Losing weight

Taking an Accurate Temperature

- The three most effective digital ways to take a baby's temperature are rectally, axillary (under the arm) and with a temporal artery thermometer. (The use of a mercury thermometer is now discouraged by the American Academy of Pediatrics.) When using the digital thermometer, be sure to follow the packaging instructions.
- The rectal method is the most accurate, since it provides a quick reading of Baby's internal temperature. The normal range for a rectal temperature is 97-99° F. If your child has a temperature 100.4 F or higher, contact your baby's doctor. While an axillary temperature is adequate, it may take longer to get an accurate reading, and that reading is usually one to two degrees lower than a rectal temperature. Therefore, if the auxiliary temperature is 99 F contact your pediatrician.
- Until a child is able to safely hold the thermometer under his tongue (approximately at age three), a rectal or axillary thermometer will be the two choices available. Always

consider the external factors that may influence your baby's temperature, such as hot weather or being overdressed. Dehydration, immunizations and teething may cause a low-grade fever of 99-100° F.

TAKING CARE OF MOM

A well-balanced diet that provides Mom's nutritional needs will help her stay strong. In addition to a healthy diet, she should continue taking prenatal vitamins throughout lactation and drink 8 ounces of water at each feeding to accommodate the production of milk. Water really is the best liquid for that; milk does not make milk, so it is not necessary for Mom to increase her normal dairy intake.

BREASTFEEDING CHALLENGES

Chapter Four, "Facts on Feeding," has a lengthy discussion on breastfeeding basics and additional information is in Appendix Four, "Monitoring Your Baby's Growth." This section highlights several difficulties that may occur with breastfeeding.

Sleepy Baby

A sleepy baby tends to nurse poorly, meaning he fails to take in adequate milk. Changing his diaper or undressing him down to his diaper might awaken him enough to help him nurse efficiently. Placing a cool, damp washcloth on his feet can arouse him out of his slumber.

Underweight Baby or a Baby that is Losing Weight

Whenever parents notice or sense their baby is not gaining weight—or is losing weight—have the baby evaluated for potential medical problems. If no underlying medical condition is detected, try supplemental formula feedings of 2-3 ounces after the baby has nursed until the weight issue is resolved.

Premature Baby

Depending on how premature your baby is and if there

are underlying conditions, your pediatrician will provide the necessary guidance regarding breastfeeding. If your baby is not able to start breastfeeding immediately, you can express or store your milk for later use with regular bottles or through specially-designed preemie bottles.

EXPRESSION OF MILK FROM THE BREAST

The reasons for expressing (withdrawing) milk from the breast range from medical necessity to comfort and convenience. The best time to pump is following the baby's feeding, particularly the first-morning feeding when Mom's milk supply is the greatest. Although milk can be expressed manually, mechanical expression is most effective.

Electric Pump:

- Wash hands thoroughly.
- Can be purchased or rented.
- Follow instructions for the type of appliance used.
- Check your local pharmacy for availability.

Hand Pump:

- Wash hands thoroughly. Support the breast by placing a hand under the breast and place pump over the areola.
- Use other hand to gently and rhythmically pump the slide or plunger.

Manual Expression:

- Wash hands thoroughly. Place fingers under the breast for support with the thumb on top.
- Compress with the thumb sliding towards the nipple (approximately 30 times per minute).

Recommendations for Proper Expression of Milk

Place expressed milk into a sterile container (plastic bags

such as Playtex™® sterile bags are preferable to glass bottles), cover, mark the time and date, and store in refrigerator. *That milk should be used within 24 hours.* If you are expressing milk for later use, follow the same procedure and place in a freezer that is 0 degrees F (the standard temperature of kitchen freezers. Check your manual to make sure your freezer is on the proper setting). You can store the milk up to six months.

To thaw breastmilk, place it in a pan of warm water and gradually increase the temperature until the milk has liquefied and is warmed sufficiently for feeding. The breastmilk will separate into layers; this is normal. Simply shake the bottle to mix it and serve immediately. (Do not let the milk sit around after thawing.) Once breastmilk is thawed, it cannot be re-frozen. Dispose of any milk remaining after the feeding since the baby's saliva breaks it down (this is true for formula as well). Reminder: Do not microwave breastmilk, since that destroys some of the infection-fighting properties in the milk.

MOM, BREASTFEEDING AND CHALLENGES

In Appendix Four, we address a number of breastfeeding challenges associated with the baby. This section will be limited to breastfeeding challenges related to Mom.

Engorged Breasts

Engorgement is most common during or right after breastmilk transitions from the initial colostrum to mature milk. It is more noticeable in moms who miss several nursing periods or if Baby is not taking all Mom is producing. Engorgement is more frequent with the first breastfed child than with subsequent children because the transition time between colostrum and mature milk seems to decrease with each child. To reduce or eliminate engorgement, make sure your baby is taking full feedings at each feeding, not skipping nursing periods or going longer then 3 hours between feedings. Mom will get relief from expressing her milk manually or by pumping. One home remedy is to take a warm shower just before feeding, but since taking eight showers a day is not practical, perhaps you can try one to two a day until the discomfort subsides.

Tender, Lumpy, or Painful Breasts

Some mothers experience breast tenderness in the days before the mature milk comes in. The baby has to suck hard to receive the colostrum, which is thicker than the mature milk that follows. A typical pattern is "suck, suck, suck, swallow." When mature milk becomes available, your baby responds with a rhythmic "suck, swallow, suck, swallow, suck, swallow." At that point, the hard sucking is reduced and the tenderness should dissipate.

Sometimes a tight-fitting bra can cause the problem, so be sure to have a properly-fitting nursing bra. Most maternity stores or hospital lactation consultants can advise you on a proper fit. Another solution is to be sure to offer both breasts at each feeding, alternating sides at the beginning of each feeding and allowing 5-10 minutes of nursing on each side to ensure the breasts are completely emptied.

Mastitis

Mastitis is an infection that affects 10 percent of nursing moms, but does not necessarily lead to the cessation of breastfeeding (consult your doctor for specifics on this matter). Bacteria enter through cracked nipples or reddened cracks in the skin or may come from a plugged milk-duct caused by a tight-fitting or underwire bra. If the bra creeps up when you lift your arms, you could be at risk for a blocked duct. Prompt attention and treatment can help keep the infection in check and bring about improvement after two days. A laboratory culture may be taken of the baby's mouth to determine if an organism such as yeast is causing the infection. For aches or fever, take a mild pain reliever such as Tylenol®. Your doctor may also prescribe antibiotics.

Yeast Infection (Candida Albicans)

"Thrush" is a yeast (or fungal infection) known as Candida Albicans. Virtually all adults test positive for Candida, and by six months of age, 90 percent of all infants test positive. A baby's immune system is normally sufficient to keep the growth of yeast in check, preventing overt symptoms; but a sick infant with a weakened immune system is vulnerable and can demonstrate the condition of oral thrush. Symptoms include white patches in the mouth that can cause problems for Baby during feeding. He becomes irritable and nursing is difficult.

A secondary problem is that oral thrush passes from Baby to Mom during breastfeeding, causing breast soreness during nursing. If you find that your baby is unwilling to feed and discover a white coating on the inside of his mouth, contact your pediatrician. The sooner this condition is treated, the sooner Baby and Mom can resume a positive nursing experience.

Plugged Duct

A tender, sore area or a lump in the breast indicates a duct may be plugged because of irregular or incomplete emptying of the milk duct, improper latching or positioning of the baby on the breast, or a poorly fitting bra. Most plugged ducts will correct themselves if taken care of quickly. Applying heat to the area before nursing to increase circulation helps unclog the duct. Maintain your nursing routine and have the baby begin nursing on the affected side first, and get adequate rest. If after 24 hours you see no improvement, or the symptoms become worse, be sure to call your doctor.

Inverted Nipples

There are three levels of nipple inversion; speak with your Ob/Gyn about the various corrective options for your case and the procedures available to assist with breastfeeding. For the mother with flat or inverted nipples, getting help early with latching on and positioning can make the difference between successful lactation and early weaning. While this condition does not pose a health risk, it can be challenging for a new mother who is working to get her baby to latch on properly. Inverted nipples do not prevent women from producing milk, but do impact the delivery of milk to the nursing baby.

Sore Nipples

Sore nipples are often the result of incorrect positioning on the breast, which causes the baby not to latch on or suckle properly. Other causes of soreness are breast engorgement, the baby latching onto the nipple only instead of both nipple and areola, improperly removing the baby from the breast, and allowing the baby to nurse too long.

The main treatment is to make sure your baby is properly positioned and latched on. You may want to rotate starting sides to distribute the nursing, possibly nursing last on the side that is sorest and slowly building up to 10 minutes on each side. Avoid using nursing pads with plastic linings. Alternate feeding positions, so the pressure from suckling does not always fall on the same part of the nipple. After nursing, allow your nipples to air dry for a few moments. Using a small amount of Vitamin E oil, lanolin, or breast cream can be helpful when applied right after nursing and does not need to be washed off until the next feeding. Mothers will also find relief when they use cotton bra pads and change them often, at least once a day or each time they become soiled through leaking milk. If pain is severe, talk to your doctor, and he or she may need to prescribe some medication.

Too Much Milk

As we noted in Chapter Six, the production of too much milk affects the cumulative balance between the foremilk and hindmilk. Babies have a set amount of foremilk and hindmilk that they need per serving. Using our example from Chapter Six, let's say your baby needs a total of 5 ounces of milk per feeding. The condition of too much milk makes more of both kinds of milk available at each feeding. Instead of taking 2 ½ ounces from one breast, the baby is taking 3, 3½ or 4 ounces. Since the baby only needs 5 ounces, when it is time to switch breasts, the baby takes just the foremilk and is satiated. Now the foremilk/hindmilk balances are off in the baby's digestive track. Because the foremilk is high in lactose but lower in fat than the hindmilk, too much lactose enters the baby's digestive system.

Three unintended consequences usually follow: First, the second breast is not getting emptied, which can lead to plugged ducts and mastitis. Second, the greater amounts of lactose can cause excessive spitting up and tummy discomfort because of gas buildup. Third, with more foremilk, Baby wakes early out of his naps, because foremilk can suppress hunger but cannot satisfy it.

To reduce the amount of milk being produced, reduce the amount of time your baby nurses at each breast. This will signal the brain to slow down on the supply. If milk is being delivered too quickly when the baby starts to nurse, pump or hand express just enough milk to slow down the flow. Do not pump the excess milk after feedings since that will encourage greater milk production.

Not Enough Milk

Poor milk production may signal poor general health, poor nutrition or inadequate fluid intake. It can also occur if Mom is particularly anxious, tense, apprehensive, or exhausted. It can also happen because Baby is receiving supplemental bottles several times a day, decreasing the number of nursing periods needed to maintain an adequate supply of milk. Here are some indicators that your baby is not receiving adequate nutrition.

- crying during and between feedings
- vigorously sucking on his hand or pacifier
- losing weight

- not producing enough urine or is constipated

If you are experiencing the problem of poor milk production, be sure to nurse your baby in a quiet area every 2½ to 3 hours, for approximately 15 minutes per side. To the extent that it is possible, try to relax during each feeding. If you are having difficulty relaxing, call your doctor and seek treatment to rule out any underlying medical issues. Try expressing milk after each feeding to see if that helps increase milk production. Electric pumps are preferable for this.

For more articles and ideas relating to taking care of Baby and Mom, please visit*www.Facebook.com/BabywiseLife*. Share your experience, be encouraged and connect with other moms.

Appendix Two

What to Expect and When

One of the great parenting myths of our day is that parents will intuitively know what to do upon the arrival of their baby. In truth, first-time parents are apt to be stressed as they learn to adjust to the overwhelming presence of a helpless infant in the home. After leaving the security of the hospital staff, those first few days and weeks are likely to be filled with uncertainty.

It may not be possible to be fully prepared as a first-time parent, because along with the arrival of the first child comes a variety of new experiences and emotions. We do believe, however, that parents are better prepared to deal with the changes a baby brings to their lives when Mom and Dad have a basic understanding of what to expect in the days following birth. This Appendix describes what usually takes place during the first three days through the first three weeks after delivery. Becoming familiar with the various expectations will spare Mom and Dad unnecessary concern.

Next to each item listed, we provide two boxes to check. As you initially read through the list before your baby arrives, place a check mark (✓) next to each item in the first row of boxes. When you have a newborn sleeping in the next room, go through the list again and check the second box. Why two boxes? Because the first time you are reading to become familiar with the subject matter, but the second time you will have a burning desire to comprehend it, driven by a heightened sensitivity for the welfare of a little life totally dependent on you.

WHAT TO EXPECT IN THE FIRST THREE DAYS

- ☐ ☐ A baby is most alert right after delivery and usually ready to nurse.
- ☐ ☐ Colostrum is a baby's first milk and present at birth.
- ☐ ☐ After a Cesarean birth, Baby is usually able to nurse soon after Mom is moved to the recovery room.
- ☐ ☐ Baby's meconium stool (dark and sticky like tar) should have passed within the first 48 hours after delivery, followed by transition stools over the next several days.
- ☐ ☐ A baby should urinate within the first 24 hours after delivery.
- ☐ ☐ Within 24-48 hours, your baby should start having wet diapers, increasing to three to five per day as Mom's milk comes in.
- ☐ ☐ Babies usually lose 7-8 ounces from their recorded birth weight within the first 24-36 hours. Your baby's hospital-discharge weight is more reflective of your baby's actual body weight and is the better base line for your baby's growth.
- ☐ ☐ One of the biggest challenges of the first 72 hours is a baby's sleepiness. Parents must keep their baby awake to take full feedings approximately every 2-3 hours.
- ☐ ☐ Follow proper umbilical-cord care and hygiene at each diaper change. If your son has been circumcised, provide the appropriate care at each diaper change.
- ☐ ☐ In these early days, be more concerned with providing your baby 8-10 good feedings every 24 hours than establishing your baby's routine or sleeping patterns.
- ☐ ☐ Remember that for now, your baby's feeding time is his waketime.

WHAT CONCERNS TO LOOK FOR IN THE FIRST THREE DAYS

- ☐ ☐ The color of Baby's skin is yellow: After the first day, newborns usually develop jaundice, which produces a yellowish hue to their skin. If that happens, a doctor will usually order a blood test to measure the level of bilirubin, which then determines the course of treatment. If the yellow tint appears after discharge from the hospital, be sure to contact your baby's doctor.
- ☐ ☐ Baby is lethargic, very sleepy or unwilling to feed: While it is common for newborns in the first week to be sleepy, it should not interfere with feeding. If you are breastfeeding, make sure your baby is properly positioned at the breast and properly latched on. Seek the experience of a lactation consultant or your doctor if you have any concerns.

WHAT TO EXPECT DURING THE FIRST THREE WEEKS

- ☐ ☐ The transition milk comes in between days three and five and by week three, mature breastmilk should be in.
- ☐ ☐ Continue to focus on full feedings.
- ☐ ☐ Monitor your baby's growth using the Healthy Baby Growth Chart in Appendix Five. By week two, the baby should have regained his birth weight or be close to it.
- ☐ ☐ The baby's stools will transition in color and consistency after the third day.
- ☐ ☐ The stools of breastfed babies tend to be softer and a lighter color than that of formula-fed babies. By five and seven days of age, a baby should have at least 3 to 5 loose yellow stools per day.
- ☐ ☐ By five to seven days, a baby should have a least 6-8 wet diapers, some saturated. Urine varies in color from nearly clear to dark yellow.

- ☐ ☐ Like adults, the color of the urine helps determine if your baby is receiving enough milk to keep him adequately hydrated. Colorless or pale-yellow urine suggests adequate hydration; darker, apple-juice-colored urine (by the end of the first week) suggests that Baby is not receiving enough milk.
- ☐ ☐ Continue providing umbilical-cord care at each diaper change until cord stump falls off. That usually happens around week two. During this time, the baby needs only a sponge bath: do not immerse him in water. Remember, if your son has been circumcised, provide the proper care with each diaper change until the circumcision is healed.
- ☐ ☐ Between ten days to three weeks, babies may have a growth spurt and require additional feedings. This may last from one to three days.
  - ☐ ☐ For a breastfed baby, feeding could be as often as every two hours (possibly extending through the night) for one to three days.
  - ☐ ☐ For a formula-fed infant, parents will notice that their baby appears hungry after consuming the normally-prepared number of ounces; or he is showing signs of hunger sooner than the next scheduled feeding. There are a couple of options to consider:
    - ☐ ☐ Add 1-2 ounces to his bottle at each feeding, allowing baby to take as much as he wants. If baby was taking 2½ oz. per feeding, make a full 4 oz. bottle and allow him to eat until full; or
    - ☐ ☐ Offer the extra feeding as Baby shows signs of hunger. When the growth spurt is over Baby will return to his normal

feed-wake-sleep routine. However, on the day following a growth spurt most babies take longer than normal naps.

- ☐ ☐ By week three, alertness should be increasing at feeding times. Between weeks three and four, your baby's waketime will begin to emerge as a separate activity apart from eating. His schedule should look something like this: feeding, burping and diaper change takes about 30+ minutes. A little bit of waketime adds another 20+ minutes. Naptime is 1½ to 2 hours.
- ☐ ☐ Not all feed-wake-sleep cycles during the day will be exactly the same length of time. That is why a range of times is provided and not *fixed* times.
- ☐ ☐ If breastfeeding, do not allow your baby to go longer than 3 hours between feedings during the first three weeks. The feed-sleep cycle should not exceed 3 to 3½ hours during the first three weeks. At night, do not allow your newborn to go more than 4 hours between feedings. (Normal feeding times usually fall between 2½ to 3 hours.)

WHAT CONCERNS TO LOOK FOR IN THE FIRST THREE WEEKS

- ☐ ☐ By 5-7 days, if your baby is not having a least 6-8 wet diapers, or not having at least 3-5 loose yellow stools per day, contact your baby's pediatrician.
- ☐ ☐ Baby is unwilling to feed.
  - ☐ ☐ If breastfeeding, make sure Baby is properly positioned at the breast, is latching on properly and that milk is being let-down. Check inside your baby's mouth for any presence of oral thrush, which is caused by the yeast Candida Albican. Signs include a milky white substance that coats the roof and side of the baby's mouth.

- ☐ ☐ If bottle feeding, make sure the nipple opening is neither too small nor too big. If too small, then Baby is sucking too hard to get the milk and may pull away. If the nipple opening is too big, the milk will come out too fast, usually causing Baby to gag and pull away. Change to appropriate size nipple.

☐ ☐ If your baby cries excessively before, during or after feedings, or if he is sleeping less than one hour and wakes up crying, call your pediatrician. Make sure you are keeping track of Baby's intake and output with the Healthy Baby Growth Chart, (Appendix Five).

There is so much more to learn and enjoy in the journey ahead. Visit us online to continue the dialogue at *www.Facebook.com/BabywiseLife*. This is a great resource for our parenting journey.

Appendix Three

Problem Solving

You feed, cuddle and bathe your baby. A diaper change here and a rattle shake there. Is this the extent of life with Baby? Only if Baby is the store-bought variety, complete with two outfits and a bottle of disappearing milk! Your baby is unlike any other. He is a complete person with complex needs and cannot be programmed according to any book or theory. Certainly, raising a baby brings an abundance of joy, yet intermingled with outstanding moments of accomplishments are the unknown challenges of parenting.

Here we explore some questions *PDF* parents commonly ask. Some of our answers are a simple summary, some refer you back to a specific text or chart, while others require additional information presented here. Do not wait for a challenging situation to arise before reading this chapter. Be proactive. Because these questions represent real-life situations, understanding them can prevent as many problems as they solve and also serve you as an excellent review of *Babywise*.

WEEK ONE

1. How soon after birth can I implement PDF?

In terms of the thought process, you begin immediately. In practice, however, you should ease yourself into the plan. To the extent that it is possible, try to relax in the early days, as you start to become acquainted with Baby and your new role as Mom. The best place to start is managing your baby's feeding times and working with your baby to take full feedings. Giving 8-10 feedings in a 24-hour period will place your baby on a predictable 3-hour routine by the end of the first week or two. Remember, do not worry about waketimes in these early days, and do not even think about nighttime sleep training until after four weeks.

2. *When my baby is brought to me for his very first feeding, how long should I let him nurse?*

Try to nurse your baby as soon as you can after birth since newborns are most alert at this time. Strive for 15 minutes per side, with a minimum of 10 minutes on each breast. This will allow for sufficient stimulation of the breasts to produce milk. If your baby wants to nurse longer during this first feeding, allow him to do so. In fact, with the first several feedings, you can go as long as the two of you are comfortable. However, be sure both breasts are stimulated at each feeding.

3. *My baby has jaundice. Should I offer water between feedings?*

Your pediatrician will direct the appropriate treatment for jaundice and use of liquid supplements. However, breastmilk is the best liquid cure for jaundice. In some cases, more frequent breastfeeding will be necessary.

4. *How do I know if my baby is getting enough food during the first week before my milk comes in?*

Check his diaper. A healthy stooling pattern is a positive indicator of adequate nutrition. During the first week, a baby's stools transition from greenish black and sticky (meconium) to a brownie-batter color and consistency. They then transition to a mustard-yellow color (a little darker for formula-fed babies). After the first week, look for 2-5 or more yellow stools each day along with 7-8 wet diapers. These indicate your baby is getting what he needs.

WEEK TWO THROUGH SEVEN

5. My baby seems to have his days and nights mixed up. He sleeps long stretches during the day and has his alert time at night. How do I fix it?

Start with a consistent time that works well for you and your family for Baby's first morning feeding. Wake your sleeping baby if necessary and work with him to take a full feeding. Feed him at regular intervals throughout the day. In the middle of the night, let him wake naturally but during the first five weeks, breastfed babies should not be allowed to sleep longer than 5 hours at night before offering a feeding.

6. My baby is fussy between 8:00 P.M. and 11.00 P.M. What's wrong?

Probably nothing! Every baby has a personal fussy time. For most, it is usually in the late afternoon or early evening. This is true for both bottle and breastfed infants. If you experience this, you are in good company; literally millions of mothers and fathers are going through the same thing at just about the same time each day. If your baby is not comforted by the baby swing, an infant seat, a sibling, Grandma or you, place him in his crib. At least there he may fall asleep. If you have a baby who becomes exceptionally and continuously fussy, he may be hungry. How is your milk supply? Go back to Chapter Four and look at the factors influencing your milk production. Review the types of foods you are eating. Hot, spicy foods or a large intake of dairy products and caffeine can contribute to a baby's fussiness.

7. My two-week-old daughter nurses on one side, then falls asleep. One hour later, she wants to eat again. What should I do?

If she is hungry, feed her, but work on keeping your baby awake to take a full feeding from both breasts. Try changing her diaper between sides, undressing her or rubbing her head and feet with a cool, damp washcloth. Do what you must to keep her awake. Then finish the task at hand: a full feeding. Keep that goal clearly in your mind. Babies learn very quickly to become snackers if you let them.

8. My three-week-old baby starts to cry one hour after his last feeding and appears hungry. I've tried to stretch his time but cannot get him to go longer. What's the problem?

Feed him, but try to find out why he is not reaching the minimum mark and start working toward it. Check your Healthy Baby Growth Chart (Appendix Five) for signs of adequate nutrition. Has he been receiving full feedings? Is he starting a growth spurt? How is your milk supply? The answers will help guide you to a workable solution.

9. My three-week-old baby is waking up after 30 minutes of naptime. Is this a nap problem or could it be something else?

There are two common reasons for this: either he needs a burp or was over-stimulated before going to sleep. If burping is the cause, get him up and gently work on releasing the bubble. If over-stimulation is the culprit, determine how to prevent this in the future. Was your baby excessively carried, bounced, played with or just kept awake too long in hopes of tiring him out? Such efforts usually backfire because babies, especially preemies, handle over-stimulation by neurologically shutting down. What appears to be sleep is not sleep at all but a self-protective neurological strategy.

10. Sometimes right after I feed my baby, he spits up what looks to be a good amount of the feeding. Should I feed him again right away?

Your baby may seem to have lost his whole meal and then some, and at three o'clock in the morning it looks even worse. Actually, the amount appears greater than its true volume. Normally another feeding is not necessary, and most babies can wait until the next routine feeding. The two most common reasons for projectile vomiting are overfeeding and doing a poor job of burping a baby. If this problem persists, it may signal a digestive problem; so be sure to contact your pediatrician.

11. Occasionally, just after I have fed, changed, and played with my baby, I will put him down for a nap and within five minutes he starts crying—hard. This is unusual for him. What should I do?

Since this is not normal behavior, it calls for your attention. He may simply have a messy diaper or need to be burped. Continue to monitor your baby to see if this is becoming a pattern. If it is, it might be the first signs of reflux, which does not always show up at birth. (See Chapter Eight.)

12. My three-week-old breastfed baby has started to sleep through the night already. Is that okay?

No! This is not acceptable for a breastfed baby because she needs the extra nourishment in these early weeks and you need the stimulation for your milk supply to be consistent. Go in and wake your baby for a feeding at least one time at night until she is six weeks old. Even at six weeks, make sure your breastfed baby does not go longer than 8 hours at night and has at least 7-8 good feedings during the day.

WEEKS EIGHT AND BEYOND

13. My baby is ten weeks old and has not yet slept through the night. What should I do to eliminate the middle-of-the-night feeding?

There are several options. First, go back and review the specific guidelines listed in Chapter Five, Managing Your Baby's Day. Are you following them? Second, do nothing for a couple of weeks because 97 percent of all *PDF* babies sleep through the night on their own by twelve weeks. Third, keep track of the exact times your baby is waking. If he is waking every night at basically the same time, he is probably waking out of habit rather than need. In this case, you may choose to help him eliminate the feeding period. Normally this takes three to five nights and is usually accompanied by some crying. Rest assured, your baby will not remember those nights and neither will you. What you will recall in days, months and years to come is a healthy, happy, well-rested baby.

14. I recently was at a family gathering and put my eight-week-old down for a nap. He began to cry, and everyone looked to see what I would do. My Aunt Martha volunteered to get the baby. I let her do it, but I felt pressured between my son needing a nap and my family wanting me to do something. What should I have done?

This answer depends on your baby's age. If Aunt Martha wants to "rescue" the baby, your three week old will probably fall asleep very comfortably in Aunt Martha's arms, and that will be fine for this one visit. When your baby is six months old, it would be better to let Aunt Martha know that her favorite nephew will be up and ready for hugs and kisses in a couple of hours in a much happier frame of mind.

15. My eight-week-old is sleeping 7-8 eight hours. Unfortunately they are the wrong 8 hours (8:00 p.m. to 4:00 a.m.). What adjustment should we make?

There is probably too much flexibility with his first feeding of the day. As this feeding time becomes consistent, everything down the line will change. It is just a matter of reworking Baby's schedule from that point forward with the goal of having 10:00 or 11:00 p.m. as the last feeding of the day. This small adjustment usually corrects the problem.

16. My baby is nine weeks old. I thought I had naps down, but suddenly, he is waking up after 45 minutes. What is the problem?

The source of the problem may be a lactation problem, a disruptive schedule, an unsettled tummy or all the above. Review the details of Chapter Six for sleep and nap recommendations.

17. My baby, at eleven weeks, extended his sleep from 8½ hours to 10 hours, but he is now waking at 5:00 a.m. for his morning feeding instead of 6:30 a.m. What should I do?

This is a common scenario, so place a checkmark next to this paragraph because you may be revisiting it early some morning. Here are three options to try. First, wait 10-15 minutes to make sure your baby is truly awake. He may be moving from an active sleep state to a deeper sleep. Second, you can feed your baby and put him back down. Awaken him at 7:00 a.m. and feed him again. Although that is less than 3 hours, the advantage is your baby is now on a normal morning routine. Third, offer a feeding at 5:00 a.m., treating it as your first feeding of the day. Then adjust the rest of the baby's morning schedule so that by early afternoon, he is back on a routine for the last and first feedings of the day being at a time you think is best for your family.

18. My baby is three months old. We recently visited relatives for a week and now, he's off schedule. How long will it take me to get him back into his regular routine?

Whenever you go on a trip, your baby is bound to get off schedule. It may be because of time-zone changes, airports or Grandma's insistence on holding him when he should be sleeping. On such rare occasions, let the relatives enjoy the baby. He will not be a baby for long. It may take a few days to get him back on schedule when you return home—along with some crying and protesting—but in three days he should be back on track.

19. My breastfed baby is thirteen weeks old. Is he ready to move to twelve hours of nighttime sleep?

At this age, a breastfed baby can extend his nighttime sleep up to 9-10 hours. The bottle-fed baby can go longer. Since breastfeeding mothers need to stay mindful of their milk production, letting your baby sleep longer than 9-10 hours at night probably will not give you enough time during the day for sufficient stimulation.

20. My baby is 3 ½ months old and is not completing his third nap. What should I do?

At this age, if your baby is getting a short third nap each day, just make sure the other two are 1½ to 2 hours long. If he sleeps 30-45 minutes for the third nap, that is enough to get him through the evening.

21. Our baby is doing well on his routine, but everything gets disrupted on Sunday morning when we drop him off at our church's newborn nursery. How can I minimize the disruption to his schedule without staying home from church for the next several months?

As noted in Chapter Five, nursery and day-care workers usually have their hands full with a number of children. Because of that fact, they cannot keep track of the different routines of each child in their care. We suggest parents leave a snack and a bottle of water, formula or breastmilk; then give the attendant the freedom to do what she thinks is best for your baby in those moments when your baby has a need that falls outside of his normal routine. When you have a well-established routine, a few hours in a nursery setting will not throw your child off. When you get home, make the appropriate adjustments.

22. My baby has been gaining weight just fine, but now at four months he is not gaining at the same rate. Is this cause for concern?

If you are seeing a steady decrease in weight gain, it might be a food or medical issue. Before checking with your doctor, rule out the food option by considering your milk supply. If you observe routine fussiness after feedings, or your baby is having difficulty going the appropriate duration between feedings, review the external stresses in your life and eliminate what you can. Are you too busy or not getting enough sleep? Are you drinking enough liquids? Is your calorie intake adequate? Are you dieting too soon? Are you following your doctor's recommendation for supplemental vitamins during lactation? Make sure you are well acquainted with Appendix Four: Monitoring Your Baby's Growth.

23. *I'm just starting Babywise with a 9-month-old. Is it too late?*

Parents who do not start out with the advantages of the *Babywise* infant-management plan may awaken to the need after their babies are six to eighteen months old and still not sleeping through the night. Is it too late for these parents? Absolutely not! If you are in this situation and desire to correct the problem, here are general and specific guidelines for establishing continuous nighttime sleep.

General Guidelines

a. Make sure you have read and understand the entire contents of this book before doing anything.
b. Do not try to make any changes while out-of-town guests or relatives are visiting. You do not need the added pressure of explaining everything you are doing.
c. Start the process of change when your baby is healthy.

Specific Guidelines

a. Work on your baby's daytime routine for the first four to five days. Keep in mind his three basic activities in the right order: feeding time, waketime and naptime. Review Chapter Five, Managing Your Baby's Day, to determine the appropriate number of feedings in a 24-hour period for your child's age. For example, a three-month-old baby should be receiving four to five feedings a day. If he is six months old, he should be receiving three meals a day with a nursing period or a bottle just before bed. If you have been rocking or nursing your baby to sleep at naptime, now is the time to eliminate that habit.

b. Review Chapter Seven, When Your Baby Cries, and be prepared for some crying. You are moving from high-comfort sleep manipulation to training in sleep skills. Initially, your baby will not like this change but it is necessary for his healthy development. The crying only means he has not yet developed the ability to settle himself. That goal is precisely what you are working toward. Be patient and consistent. For some parents, success comes after one night; for others, it comes after two weeks. The average is three to five days. Continue to think about and look toward long-term benefits. Your proactive response is best not only for your baby but also for your entire family.

SUMMARY

Retraining is always more difficult than training correctly from the start, but parents who love their babies give them what they need—and young children need a good night's sleep! Moms who have seen their babies make the transition from sleepless nights to peaceful sleep report that their daytime disposition changes dramatically as well. They are happier, more content and definitely more manageable. We trust this will be the case with your baby as well. For more helpful information, connect with us at <u>*www.Facebook.com/BabywiseLife*</u>.

Appendix Four

Monitoring Your Baby's Growth

One of many advantages of parent-directed feeding is the success mothers have with breastfeeding. Knowing your baby's nutritional needs are being met in an orderly fashion provides greater confidence. While confidence is a positive thing, do not become complacent when it comes to monitoring your baby's growth.

This is something that is important to us, and should be to you. Your baby's life depends on it! Knowing what to expect in the first week and knowing what nutritional indicators to look for can make all the difference in the world, when it comes to your sense of confidence and baby's welfare. These indicators provide Mom with guidance and feedback on how well she and her baby are doing. They confirm that things are going well and they warn of any condition that needs your immediate attention. Anytime you notice unhealthy indicators, call your pediatrician and report your objective findings.

Included in the next Appendix are age-related *Healthy Baby Growth Charts,* designed to assist you in your daily evaluation. The first is designed specifically for week one; the second chart covers weeks two through four, and the third chart covers weeks five and beyond. Using these charts will provide important benchmarks signaling healthy or unhealthy growth patterns. What are the indicators that Mom and Dad should be looking for? Let's review them.

WEEK ONE: HEALTHY GROWTH INDICATORS

1. Under normal circumstances, it takes only a few minutes for your baby to adjust to life outside the womb. His eyes will open and he will begin to seek food. Bring your baby to breast as soon as it is possible, and certainly try to do so within the first hour and a half after birth. One of the first and most basic positive indicators is your baby's willingness and desire to nurse.

2. It is natural to wonder and to even be a little anxious during the first few postpartum days. How do you know if your baby is getting enough food to live on? The release of the first milk, colostrum, is a second important encouraging indicator. In the simplest terms, colostrum is a protein concentrate ideally suited for your baby's nutritional and health needs. One of the many benefits of colostrum is its effect on your baby's first bowel movement. It helps trigger the passage of the meconium, your baby's first stools. Newborn stools in the first week transition from the meconium stool to a brownie-batter transition stool to a mustard-yellow stool. The three to five soft or liquid yellow stools by the fourth or fifth day are totally breastmilk stools and a healthy sign that your baby is getting enough nutrition. A bottle-fed baby will pass firmer, light brown to golden or clay-colored stools that have an odor similar to adult stools.

3. During the first week, frequent nursing is necessary for two reasons: first, your baby needs the colostrum and second, frequent nursing is required to establish lactation. Nursing every 2½ to 3-hours and a minimum of eight times a day are two more positive indicators to consider.

4. Just bringing your baby to breast does not mean your baby is nursing efficiently. There is a time element involved. In those early days, most babies nurse between 30 and 45 minutes. If your baby is sluggish or sleepy all the time or not nursing more than a total of ten minutes, this may be an unhealthy indicator.

5. As your baby works at taking the colostrum, you will hear him swallow. A typical pattern is suck, suck, suck, then swallow. When mature milk becomes available, your baby responds with a rhythmic suck, swallow, suck, swallow, suck, swallow. You should not hear a clicking sound nor see dimpled cheeks. A clicking sound and dimpled cheeks during nursing are two indicators that your baby is not sucking efficiently. He is sucking his own tongue, not the breast. If you hear clicking, remove baby from the breast and then relatch him.

When relatching wait for a wide open mouth. Look for lips to be flared out like fish lips. Use a finger to gently curl out the top lip if needed. Try gentle downward pressure on the baby's chin to draw out the bottom lip. If it does not resolve with practice have it checked by a Lactation Consultant or your pediatrician. (This could be a potential tongue or lip tie.)

Week One Healthy Growth Indicators

1. Your baby goes to the breast and nurses.
2. Your baby is nursing a minimum of eight times in 24-hour.
3. Your baby is nursing over fifteen minutes at each nursing period.
4. You can hear your baby swallowing milk.
5. Your baby has passed his first stool called meconium. (Since the passage of the meconium is one of the "well baby" markers of a newborn, most hospitals will not release a baby if this stool has not passed within the first 24 hours. Failure to pass the meconium stool may signal an intestinal obstruction.)
6. Your baby's stooling pattern progresses from meconium (greenish black) to brownie batter transition stools to yellow stools by the fourth or fifth day. An increased stooling pattern is a positive sign your baby is getting enough milk.
7. Within 24-48 hours, your baby starts having wet diapers increasing each day to five to six by day five.

Unhealthy Growth Indicators for Week One

1. Your baby is not showing any desire to nurse or has a very weak suck.
2. Your baby fails to nurse eight times in a 24-hour period.
3. Your baby tires quickly at the breast and cannot sustain at least fifteen minutes at the breast.
4. Your baby continually falls asleep at the breast before taking a full feeding.
5. You hear a clicking sound accompanied by dimpled cheeks during nursing.
6. Your baby's stooling pattern is not progressing to yellow stools within a week's time.
7. Your baby has not produced a wet any diapers within 24 hours of birth.

At this point, please turn to the back of the book to look at Chart One. Review it and remember to take the book with you to the hospital. Make additional copies of the charts for your own use or share them with a friend.

WEEKS TWO THROUGH FOUR: HEALTHY GROWTH INDICATORS

After the first week, some of the healthy growth indicators begin to change. Here is the check list for the next three weeks.

Healthy Growth Indicators for Weeks Two through Four

1. Your baby is nursing at least eight times a day.
2. Your baby has two to five or more yellow stools daily during the next three weeks. (This number will probably decrease after the first month.)
3. Your baby should start to have six to eight wet diapers a day (some saturated).
4. Your baby's urine is clear (not yellow).
5. Your baby has a strong suck, you see milk on the corners of his mouth, and you can hear an audible swallow.
6. You are noticing increased signs of alertness during your baby's waketime.

7. Your baby is gaining weight and growing in length. We recommend your baby be weighed within a week or two after birth. Baby should regain birth weight by day fourteen.

Unhealthy Indicators for Weeks Two through Four

1. Your baby is not getting eight feedings a day.
2. Your baby in the first month has small, scant, and infrequent stools.
3. Your baby does not have the appropriate amount of wet diapers.
4. Your baby's urine is concentrated and bright yellow.
5. Your baby has a weak or nonproductive suck, or you cannot hear him swallowing.
6. Your baby is sluggish or slow to respond to stimulus and does not sleep between feedings.
7. Your baby is not gaining weight or growing in length. Your doctor will direct you in the best strategy to correct this problem.

WEEKS FIVE AND ABOVE: HEALTHY GROWTH INDICATORS

The major difference between the first month indicators and the weeks to follow are the stooling patterns. After the first month, your baby's stooling pattern will change. He may pass only one large stool a day or pass one as infrequently as one in every three to five days. Every baby is different. Any concerns regarding elimination should be directed to your pediatrician.

Parents are responsible for seeing that their baby's health and nutritional needs are recognized and met. For your peace of mind and your baby's health, we recommend regular visits with your pediatrician and use of the charts included at the end of the book to monitor and record your baby's progress. Any two consecutive days of deviation from what is listed as normal should be reported to your pediatrician.

If you make copies of the charts, post them in a convenient location such as on the refrigerator, above the crib, or any location that will serve as a convenient reminder. If your baby exhibits any of the unhealthy growth indicators, notify your pediatrician and have your baby weighed.

Weight-Gain Concerns

With the conservative practice of *PDF*, weight gain will be steady and continuous. We routinely monitor the progress of *PDF* babies and continue to find wonderful results. In 1997, our retrospective studies tracked and compared the weight gain of 200 *PDF* infants (group A) and 200 demand-fed infants (group B). Pertinent growth information (weight gain and length) was taken directly from the patient charts of four pediatric practices.

The study's purpose was to determine if faster weight gain can be attributed to a particular method of breastfeeding (routine or demand). The weight and length of each infant was charted at birth, weeks 1 and 2; months 1, 2, 4, 6, 9 and at 1 year. Comparisons were made between five weight groups: babies born weighing between 6.50 and 7.0 lbs, 7.1 and 7.50 lbs, 7.51 and 8.0 lbs, 8.1 and 8.50 lbs, and 8.51 and 9.0 lbs.

Two methods of analysis were used to compare growth: weight gain ratios (comparing weight gained at each visit as a percentage of birth weight) and Body Mass Index (BMI). The BMI index is derived by dividing the weight expressed in kilograms, by the length (height), expressed in meters squared.

The rationale for using BMI was an attempt to obtain a more uniform basis of comparison than a simple linear contrast. Using absolute body weight alone as a comparative tool, does not embody any reference to the stature of the baby. However, an analysis using BMI allows for a more meaningful comparative study of babies with different birth weights and statures.

MAJOR CONCLUSIONS

One: While there was no significant difference between the two groups, group A (*PDF* babies) gained weight slightly faster than group B at each weight category.

Two: Even when group A began sleeping 7-8 hours at night, there was no significant change in weight-gain performance.

Three: While breastfeeding initially was the preferred method for both sets of parents, group B moms gave up breastfeeding significantly sooner than group A.

You can take comfort in the fact that a basic routine will not detract from a proper, healthy weight gain. What it will do is facilitate breastfeeding success. Even low-birth weight babies do well on a conservative routine. Although some newborns start off at the low end of the national norms, they continue to gain weight in proportion to the genetic potential for stature inherited from their parents. That is, smaller parents usually give birth to smaller babies, thus weight gain will usually be proportionately less.

When you add the benefits of healthy sleep patterns and a good night's sleep for both parents, the greater benefits of *PDF* become obvious to the user and beneficial to the baby. One note of caution: if you have a low-weight-gain baby, always seek your physician's specific recommendations as to how often your baby should be fed.

NORMAL WEIGHT-GAIN GUIDE

Birth to Two Weeks:

Approximate average: Regain birth weight plus.

Two Weeks to Three Months:

Approximate average: Two pounds per month or 1 ounce per day.

Four to Six Months:

Approximate average: One pound per month or ½ ounce per day. (Doubles his birth weight by six months.)

One Year:
Approximate average: Two and a half to three times his birth weight.

BABIES WHO FAIL TO THRIVE

There is a difference between *slow weight gain* and *failure to thrive.* With slow weight gain, weight gain is slow but consistent. Failure to thrive describes an infant who continues to lose weight after ten days of life, does not regain his or her birth weight by three weeks of age, or gains at an unusually slow rate beyond the first month. It is estimated that in the United States, more than two hundred thousand babies a year experience failure to thrive. The cause can be attributed to either mother or child.

Mother-Related Causes

Here are matters specific to mothers that can contribute to slow or no weight gain:

1. *Improper nursing technique.* Many women fail at breastfeeding because the baby is not positioned properly on the breast. As a result, he or she latches on only to the nipple and not to all or much of the areola. The end result is a hungry baby.

2. *Nature or lifestyle.* Insufficient milk production can be a result of nature (insufficient breast-milk storage capacity or hormones) or a mother's life-style (not getting enough rest or liquids). The mother simply does not produce enough milk, or in some cases, milk of high enough quality. If you suspect this is the case, try a) using a breast pump to see what quantity of milk is being produced; and b) to discover if your baby will take any formula after he has been at your breast for the proper amount of time. Report your findings to your pediatrician.

3. *Poor release of milk.* This indicates a problem with the moth-

er's let-down reflex. Contact your pediatrician or lactation consultant for help.

4. *Feeding too frequently.* There is an irony here because one would think that many feedings ensure adequate weight gain. Not necessarily! In some cases a mother can be worn out by too many ineffective feedings. When we first met Jeffrey, he was six weeks old and had gained only one pound. His mom offered him the breast each time he cried, approximately every 1 to 1½ hours. Jeffrey was properly latched on to his fatigued and frustrated mother. Although he was failing to thrive, the only counsel this mother received from her "Board Certified Lactation Consultant" was to feed more often. To further her exhaustion, she was told to carry Jeffrey in a sling. We immediately placed Jeffrey's mother on a 3-hour routine. To improve Jeffrey's poor health, he was given a formula supplement. Within a few days, the starving child started to gain weight. After just a week, he was sleeping through the night. Jeffrey's mother successfully breastfed his subsequent siblings on the *PDF* plan with no weight-gain problems. As a footnote to Jeffrey's story, the lactation advice offered should not be construed as a judgement on all consultants, but it does serve as a warning, that if you hear something that does not sound right, get a second opinion.

5. *Feeding too infrequently.* This problem can be attributed to either hyperscheduling or demand-feeding. The mother who insists on watching the clock to the minute lacks confidence in decision-making. The clock is in control, not the parent. The hyperschedulist insists on a strict schedule, often nursing her baby no sooner than every 4 hours. Enslavement to the clock is almost as great an evil as a mother who is in bondage to thoughtless emotions. Another side to the problem of infrequency is that some demand-

fed babies demand too little food. As a result, the mother's breast is not sufficiently stimulated for adequate milk production. Routine feedings with a time limitation between feedings eliminates this problem. That is why Neonatal Intensive Care Units advocate feeding routine, with feeding times determined by baby's healthy growth patterns.

6. *Not monitoring growth signs*. Many moms simply fail to notice their baby's healthy and unhealthy growth indicators. The healthy baby growth chart will assist you with this vital task. A common mistake made during the third and fourth months is to assume that just because your baby has done well up to this point, he probably will not have any problems in the future. That is not always the case. You must continue to monitor your baby's growth throughout his first year of life.

7. *Physical nurturing, holding, and cuddling.* The lack of these gestures can impact a child's ability to thrive. It is important that moms cuddle, hold, and talk to their babies frequently throughout the day. Your routine will help provide these periods, but Mom should not be the only one cuddling the child. Dad, older siblings, Grandma, and Grandpa are some of your baby's favorite people. More people, more love.

8. *Pushing too hard or too fast into the next milestone*. As we emphasized in Chapter 5, a mother cannot arbitrarily decide to drop a feeding or a nap, unless her baby has the physical *capacity* and *ability* to make the adjustment. The same warning applies here. Be careful not to compromise your baby's nutrition by pushing your baby ahead of his developmental schedule. For example, some mothers fail to notice the warning indicators of inadequate nutrition, because they are overly focused on extending nighttime sleep. If your baby is routinely waking 30 to 45 minutes into his nap, it may have more to do with inadequate nutrition

or lactation than the start of poor sleep habits.

Infant-Related Causes

Slow weight gain or an absence of weight gain also may be directly related to your infant. Here are several possibilities:

1. *Weak sucking.* In this case, the child does not have the coordination or the strength to suck properly, remain latched on, or activate the let-down reflex. As a result, the baby receives the low-calorie foremilk but not the high-calorie hindmilk.

2. *Improper sucking.* This can result from a number of different conditions:

   Tongue thrusting: When on the breast, baby thrusts his tongue forward and pushes the nipple out of his mouth.

   Protruding tongue: This condition is described as the tongue forming a hump in the mouth, interfering with successful latching on.

   Tongue-Tie: A condition at birth that restricts the tongues range of motion. This is the result of tissue holding the tongue to the floor of the month.

   Lip-Tie: This condition is the result of shortened tissue behind the upper lip, preventing the upper lip from moving freeing.

   Tongue sucking: The infant suckles on his own tongue.

3. *An underlying medical problem.* A weak or laborious suck (for example, one in which the child tires after a few minutes of nursing and gives up) can be a symptom of cardiac or neurological failing. If you have any such concerns, contact your pediatrician immediately.

WHAT YOU NEED TO KNOW ABOUT LACTATION CONSULTANTS

Even with all the classes we take, the plans we make and books we read, sometimes nursing just does not go well. It can be very frustrating in those first few days or weeks. There you are, holding a crying, wiggling, red-faced (but cute) little bundle who refuses to nurse, and all your interventions seem to be of no avail.

You may need help from a lactation consultant. These are women trained in helping mom's with breastfeeding techniques. Your pediatrician's office, hospital, or clinic will often have a consultant on staff or can refer you to one. Most consultants are "board certified." This certification represents the highest level of achievement for this profession.

However, we offer this clarifying word. The title "Board Certified" is not the same thing as being "Licensed by the State," as is the case with medical professionals such as nurses and doctors, nor does it always guarantee the advice rendered will always be the best for you or your baby. While the vast majority of consultants provide excellent, helpful guidance relating the practical mechanics of breastfeeding, there are some who allow their own parenting bias to cloud their lactation advice. For this small group we are providing a few red flags to look out for.

Red Flags

Be cautious of any consultant who instructs you to go against your pediatrician's medical guidance. Notify your pediatrician about the advice received, or send your concerns to your State and local health departments. Be equally concerned with any consultant that advises something that the American Academy of Pediatrics expressly warns against, such as co-sleeping with your baby. Likewise, if you are receiving more parenting advice from the consultant than breastfeeding mechanics, or if you are given any advice that sounds extreme, consider looking elsewhere for help.

What Consultants Look For

If you can, schedule your initial visit near a feeding time. A consultant usually will want to observe the baby nursing. She will also weigh the infant and check to see that his suckle is correct. Next, a history will be taken, including questions about the length of labor, birthing process, birth weight of the baby, your diet, how often you are nursing the baby, and more. The information logged on your healthy baby growth chart is useful to the consultant. It provides an overall picture of how your infant is doing.

When you do find the right consultant, openly share actual feeding times and precisely what you are doing. Although parenting philosophies will differ, any technical lactation intervention is applicable, whether you demand-feed or use a routine. If you hear something that does not sound right or extreme, consider getting a second opinion.

In some cases, intervention and correction are immediate. In others, such as with those infants who have a disorganized or a dysfunctional suckle, retraining the infant to suckle correctly will take some time and patience on your part. Depending on the circumstance, the lactation consultant might suggest using devices such as a syringe (minus the needle), finger-feeding, or a supplemental feeding device to help your infant learn to nurse. Sometimes these are effective; other times they are not. They also can be time-consuming to use. Discuss the choices with your husband and make your decision together. Should you use a device, reevaluate its effectiveness at some point.

Breastfeeding proficiency is usually a matter of standard review in childbirth classes. For additional help, consider taking a breastfeeding class at your local hospital or renting a how-to video. You can attend a class and learn proper techniques of breastfeeding without accepting the instructor's personal parenting philosophies that sometimes accompany such classes. Remember to keep the issue of nursing in balance. Going the "extra mile" to correct a nursing difficulty or deciding to stop and bottle-feed instead is not a positive or negative reflection on your mothering. What is important is that your husband and you decide what is best for your baby. No one else can make that decision but you and your husband.

Finally, be aware that those who practice independently tend to have higher fees than those who are affiliated with a medical practice. Check with your insurance company to find out if the cost is covered under your plan.

INSUFFICIENT MILK PRODUCTION

Regardless of which feeding philosophy you follow, you cannot add to what nature has left out. The anxiety created by the fear of failure is itself a contributor to milk deficiency. Because so much guilt is placed on mothers who are not successful at breastfeeding, many of them go to extremes to become milk-sufficient.

In most cultures, five percent of nursing mothers during peacetime and up to ten percent during wartime, will not produce enough milk to meet their infant's nutritional needs. Some mothers may initially be milk-sufficient but become insufficient by the third month. This sometimes happens even though baby is cooperative and sucking frequently and mom is using correct nursing techniques, receiving adequate food and rest, and has sufficient support from her husband and family.

We want you to be successful right from the start. The first month is the most important time to establish a healthy milk supply. Here is a quick review:

- Feed frequently, at least 8 times in 24 hours.
- Respond to feeding cues, no more than 3 hours apart.
- Work on getting full feedings because an empty breast fills faster and better than partially emptied breasts.
- Limit pacifier use and bottles in the first month.

IF YOU QUESTION YOUR MILK SUPPLY

If at any time you question the adequacy of your milk supply, observe routine fussiness after every feeding, or your baby is having difficulty going the appropriate duration between feedings, review the external stresses in your life. Eliminate what you can. This is true whether baby is four weeks old or four months old.

Ask yourself the following: Are you too busy or not getting enough sleep? Are you drinking enough liquids? Is your intake of calories adequate? Are you dieting too soon, or are you on birth control pills? Are you following your doctor's recommendation for supplemental vitamins during lactation? Also consider the technical aspects associated with feeding. Is the baby positioned properly and latched on correctly? Is your baby taking a full feeding from both breasts?

1. *If you question your milk supply in the first two months:* for a baby between three and eight weeks old, consider feeding on a strict 2½-hour routine for five to seven days. If your milk production increases (as demonstrated by the baby becoming more content and sleeping better), work your way back to the 3-hour minimum. If no improvement comes, work back up to 3 hours with the aid of a formula complement for the benefit of your baby and your own peace of mind.

2. *If you question your milk supply in the fourth month, the same basic principles apply to this age category.* If your baby is between four and six months of age and you question your milk supply, try adding a couple of feedings to your daytime routine. One of our mothers, also a pediatrician, felt she was losing her milk supply at four months. She did two things. She added a fifth feeding to her day, and she stopped dieting. In less than one week her milk supply was back to normal.

Other mothers find success by returning to a fairly tight 3-hour schedule. Once their milk supply returns to normal, they gradually return to their previous routine. If no improvement comes after five to seven days, consider a formula complement. Adding a few extra feedings during the day is not a setback in your parenting but necessary to insure a healthy balance between breastfeeding and the related benefits of *PDF*.

THE FOUR-DAY TEST

You may also want to consider the four-day test. This involves offering a complementary feeding of one to two ounces of formula after each nursing period. Then, express your milk with an electric breast pump ten minutes per side. (Manual pumps are not effective for this purpose.) Keep track of how much extra you are producing. If your milk is plentiful, then store it and use for the next feeding in place of formula. This will also tell you that the problem lies with your baby. He or she is either not latching on properly or is a "lazy nurser." If your milk supply increases as a result of pumping, which will be indicated either by milk expressed or by your baby not wanting the complementary feeding, then return to breastfeeding only, maintaining a 3-hour routine.

If additional stimulation from breast pumping does not increase your milk supply, and if you have reviewed all the external factors and found them compatible with nursing, then you may be among the five percent of moms who cannot provide a sufficient milk supply. Are you ready to give it up? Before you say "that's me" and quit for good, consider calling your pediatrician for advice. Ask if he or she knows of an older mother in the practice who was able to reverse this situation. You may also be referred to a lactation consultant. Remember, different opinions abound. Learn and discern what is best for your family.

For additional tools and strategies related to baby care and healthy growth, please visit www.Facebook.com/BabywiseLife.

Appendix Five

Healthy Baby Growth Charts

Signs of Adequate Nutrition

Chart One—Week One

It is important to monitor your baby's growth when breastfeeding to assure your baby is receiving adequate nutrition. There are a number of objective indicators of healthy growth to stay mindful of. Healthy signs of growth during the first week of life include:

1. Your baby goes to the breast and nurses.
2. Your baby is nursing a minimum of eight times in 24-hour.
3. Your baby is nursing over fifteen minutes at each nursing period.
4. You can hear your baby swallowing milk.
5. Your baby has passed his first stool called meconium. (Since the passage of the meconium is one of the "well baby" markers of a newborn, most hospitals will not release a baby if this stool has not passed within the first 24 hours. Failure to pass the meconium stool may signal an intestinal obstruction.)
6. Your baby's stooling pattern progresses from meconium (greenish black) to brownie batter transition stools to yellow stools by the fourth or fifth day. An increased stooling pattern is a positive sign your baby is getting enough milk.
7. Within 24-48 hours, your baby starts having wet diapers increasing each day to five to six by day five.

Unhealthy growth indicators for the first week.

1. Your baby is not showing any desire to nurse or has a very weak suck.
2. Your baby fails to nurse eight times in a 24-hour period.
3. Your baby tires quickly at the breast and cannot sustain at least 15 minutes of nursing.
4. Your baby continually falls asleep at the breast before taking a full feeding.
5. You hear a clicking sound accompanied by dimpled cheeks while baby is nursing.
6. Your baby's stooling pattern is not progressing to yellow stools within a week's time.
7. Your baby has not produced a wet any diapers within 24 hours of birth.

Using the chart to keep track of your baby's vital health indicators can make the difference between healthy and unhealthy growth. Feel free to make copies of the chart for your personal use, or to give to a friend. Place it in a convenient location (on a refrigerator, above the crib, etc.). Add the appropriate (√) mark or letter designated for each occurrence. For example, if your baby nurses nine times on day two, then there should be nine checks on that day. If your baby passes his first meconium stool on the second day, then place an "M" on that day. Knowing what to expect and measuring results will get you and your baby off to a great start. For additional charts, visit us at *www.Facebook.com/BabywiseLife.*

HEALTHY BABY GROWTH CHART: Chart One Week 1

Birth Weight ______________lb. /oz. Birth Length ______________inches

HEALTHY GROWTH INDICATORS	DAY 1	DAY 2	DAY 3	DAY 4	DAY 5	DAY 6	DAY 7
Place a check (√) for each feeding in a 24 hour period. (Minimum of 8 feedings a day.)							
Place a check (√) for each nursing period of 15 or more minutes in length.							
Place a "M" for the first stool (Meconium) and a "T" for each brownie battered transition stool.							
Place a "Y" to record each yellow stool. (Milk stools should appear by the 4th or 5th day.)							
Place a check (√) for each wet diaper. (Wet diapers should start to appear by 48 hours or sooner.)							

7–10 days: Weight ______________lb. /oz. Length ______________inches

Any two consecutive days of deviation from what is listed as normal should be reported immediately to your pediatrician.

Signs of Adequate Nutrition

Chart Two—Weeks Two through Four

After the first week, some of the healthy growth indicators begin to change. The next chart represents healthy baby growth indicators to monitored over the next three weeks. Please note the changes.

Here is the checklist for the next three weeks.

1. Your baby is nursing at least eight times a day.
2. Your baby over the next three weeks has two to five or more yellow stools daily. (This number will probably decrease after the first month.)
3. Your baby should start to have six to eight wet diapers a day, some saturated.
4. Your baby's urine is clear, not yellow.
5. Your baby has a strong suck, you see milk, and you can hear an audible swallow.
6. You are noticing increased signs of alertness during your baby's waketime.
7. Your baby is gaining weight and growing in length.

Unhealthy growth indicators are:

1. Your baby is not getting eight feedings a day.
2. Your baby has small, scant, and infrequent stools.
3. Your baby does not have the appropriate number of wet diapers given his age.
4. Your baby's urine is concentrated and bright yellow.
5. Your baby has a weak or tiring suck and you cannot hear him swallow.
6. Your baby is sluggish or slow to respond to stimulus, and does not sleep between feedings.
7. Your baby is not gaining weight or growing in length. Your doctor will direct you in the best strategy to correct this problem.

Any two consecutive days of deviation from what is listed above as normal should be reported immediately to your pediatrician. Using the chart to keep track of your baby's vital health indicators can make the difference between healthy and unhealthy growth. If you wish make copies of the chart and place it in a convenient location (on a refrigerator, above the crib, etc.). For your assurance record the results with a (√) mark for each occurrence of each healthy indicator. For example, six wet diapers on Monday should have six checks in the appropriate box. Knowing what to expect and measuring the expected results against the actual will provide the necessary security and confidence that your baby is doing fine. Keep in mind, more helpful resources and support can be found at *www.Facebook.com/BabywiseLife*.

HEALTHY BABY GROWTH CHART: Chart Two Weeks 2–4

Summary of Each Day

HEALTHY GROWTH INDICATORS	MON	TUE	WED	THU	FRI	SAT	SUN
Place a check (√) for each feeding in a 24-hour period. (Minimum of 8.)							
Place a check (√) for each wet diaper per day with clear urine. (Norm per day: 5 to 7.)							
Place a check (√) for each wet diaper with yellow concentrated urine. (Norm per day: 0.)							
Place a check (√) for each yellow stool. (For the first month, 2 to 5 or more, per day.)							

Any two consecutive days of deviation from what is listed as normal should be reported immediately to your pediatrician.

HEALTHY BABY GROWTH CHART: Chart Two Weeks 2–4

HEALTHY GROWTH INDICATORS	Summary of Each Day						
	MON	TUE	WED	THU	FRI	SAT	SUN
Place a check (√) for each feeding in a 24-hour period. (Minimum of 8.)							
Place a check (√) for each wet diaper per day with clear urine. (Norm per day: 5 to 7.)							
Place a check (√) for each wet diaper with yellow concentrated urine. (Norm per day: 0.)							
Place a check (√) for each yellow stool. (For the first month, 2 to 5 or more, per day.)							

Any two consecutive days of deviation from what is listed as normal should be reported immediately to your pediatrician.

HEALTHY BABY GROWTH CHART: Chart Two Weeks 2–4

Summary of Each Day

HEALTHY GROWTH INDICATORS	MON	TUE	WED	THU	FRI	SAT	SUN
Place a check (√) for each feeding in a 24-hour period. (Minimum of 8.)							
Place a check (√) for each wet diaper per day with clear urine. (Norm per day: 5 to 7.)							
Place a check (√) for each wet diaper with yellow concentrated urine. (Norm per day: 0.)							
Place a check (√) for each yellow stool. (For the first month, 2 to 5 or more, per day.)							

Any two consecutive days of deviation from what is listed as normal should be reported immediately to your pediatrician.

Signs of Adequate Nutrition

Chart Three—Weeks Five through Ten Weeks

This third chart differs from the second only in the number of stools eliminated. Basically the rest of the chart is the same. Continue to monitor your baby's growth, especially after your baby starts sleeping through the night.

Here is the checklist for the next six weeks.

1. Your baby is nursing at least seven to eight times a day.
2. Your baby's stooling pattern again changes. Your baby may have several small stools or one large one. He may have several a day or one every couple of days.
3. Your baby should have six to eight wet diapers a day, some saturated.
4. Your baby's urine is clear, not yellow.
5. Your baby has a strong suck, you see milk, and you can hear an audible swallow.
6. You are seeing increasing signs of alertness during your baby's waketime.
7. Your baby is gaining weight and growing in length.

Unhealthy growth indicators are:

1. Your baby is not getting a minimum of seven feedings a day.
2. Your baby does not have the appropriate number of wet diapers given his age.
3. Your baby's urine is concentrated and bright yellow.
4. Your baby has a weak or tiring suck and you cannot hear him swallow.
5. Your baby is sluggish or slow to respond to stimulus, and does not sleep between feedings.
6. Your baby is not gaining weight or growing in length. Your doctor will direct you in the best strategy to correct this problem.

Any two consecutive days of deviation from what is listed above as normal should be reported immediately to your pediatrician. Using the chart to keep track of your baby's vital health indicators can make the difference between healthy and unhealthy growth. If you wish, make copies of the chart and place it in a convenient location (on a refrigerator, above the crib, etc.). For your assurance, record the results with a (√) mark for each occurrence of each healthy indicator. For example, six wet diapers on Monday should have six checks in the appropriate box. Knowing what to expect and measuring the expected results against the actual will provide you security and confidence as your baby grows.

For more tools and strategies related to care and healthy growth visit us at *www.Facebook.com/BabywiseLife.*

HEALTHY BABY GROWTH CHART: Chart Three Weeks 5–10

	Summary of Each Day						
HEALTHY GROWTH INDICATORS	MON	TUE	WED	THU	FRI	SAT	SUN
Place a check (√) for each feeding. (Minimum should be 7-8 in a 24-hour period.)							
Place a check (√) for each wet diaper per day with clear urine (Norm per day: 5 to 7.)							
Place a check (√) for each wet diaper with yellow concentrated urine. (Norm per day: 0.)							
Place a check (√) for each stool per day.							

Any two consecutive days of deviation from what is listed as normal should be reported immediately to your pediatrician.

HEALTHY BABY GROWTH CHART: Chart Three Weeks 5–10

Summary of Each Day

HEALTHY GROWTH INDICATORS	MON	TUE	WED	THU	FRI	SAT	SUN
Place a check (√) for each feeding. (Minimum should be 7-8 in a 24-hour period.)							
Place a check (√) for each wet diaper per day with clear urine (Norm per day: 5 to 7.)							
Place a check (√) for each wet diaper with yellow concentrated urine. (Norm per day: 0.)							
Place a check (√) for each stool per day.							

Any two consecutive days of deviation from what is listed as normal should be reported immediately to your pediatrician.

HEALTHY BABY GROWTH CHART: Chart Three Weeks 5–10

HEALTHY GROWTH INDICATORS	MON	TUE	WED	THU	FRI	SAT	SUN
	Summary of Each Day						
Place a check (√) for each feeding. (Minimum should be 7-8 in a 24-hour period.)							
Place a check (√) for each wet diaper per day with clear urine (Norm per day: 5 to 7.)							
Place a check (√) for each wet diaper with yellow concentrated urine. (Norm per day: 0.)							
Place a check (√) for each stool per day.							

Any two consecutive days of deviation from what is listed as normal should be reported immediately to your pediatrician.

HEALTHY BABY GROWTH CHART: Chart Three Weeks 5–10

Summary of Each Day

HEALTHY GROWTH INDICATORS	MON	TUE	WED	THU	FRI	SAT	SUN
Place a check (√) for each feeding. (Minimum should be 7-8 in a 24-hour period.)							
Place a check (√) for each wet diaper per day with clear urine (Norm per day: 5 to 7.)							
Place a check (√) for each wet diaper with yellow concentrated urine. (Norm per day: 0.)							
Place a check (√) for each stool per day.							

Any two consecutive days of deviation from what is listed as normal should be reported immediately to your pediatrician.

HEALTHY BABY GROWTH CHART: Chart Three Weeks 5–10

Summary of Each Day

HEALTHY GROWTH INDICATORS	MON	TUE	WED	THU	FRI	SAT	SUN
Place a check (√) for each feeding. (Minimum should be 7-8 in a 24-hour period.)							
Place a check (√) for each wet diaper per day with clear urine (Norm per day: 5 to 7.)							
Place a check (√) for each wet diaper with yellow concentrated urine. (Norm per day: 0.)							
Place a check (√) for each stool per day.							

Any two consecutive days of deviation from what is listed as normal should be reported immediately to your pediatrician.

HEALTHY BABY GROWTH CHART: Chart Three Weeks 5–10

HEALTHY GROWTH INDICATORS	Summary of Each Day: MON	TUE	WED	THU	FRI	SAT	SUN
Place a check (√) for each feeding. (Minimum should be 7-8 in a 24-hour period.)							
Place a check (√) for each wet diaper per day with clear urine (Norm per day: 5 to 7.)							
Place a check (√) for each wet diaper with yellow concentrated urine. (Norm per day: 0.)							
Place a check (√) for each stool per day.							

Any two consecutive days of deviation from what is listed as normal should be reported immediately to your pediatrician.

Chapter Endnotes

Chapter One

1. See the collaborating work of Dr. John Medina. Dr. Medina is a developmental molecular biologist specializing in the genes involved in human brain development. He is the author of the *Brain Rules* and *Brain Rules for Baby.* (Pear Press 2010)

Chapter Two

1. Dr. Rupert Rogers wrote on the problems of breastfeeding during the 1930s and 1940s. He told mothers to be old-fashioned. What did he mean by that? He said to go back to nursing periods arranged as follows: 6:00 A.M., 9:00 A.M., Noon, 3:00 P.M., 6:00 P.M., 10:00 P.M., and once when the baby wakes in the night. Although that type of feeding was a schedule, it was not referred to as such. The term "schedule" referred to a nursing technique more than a routine. *Mother's Encyclopedia* (New York: The Parents Institute, Inc., 1951), p. 122.
2. Ribble, Margaret, *The Right of Infants* (New York: Columbia University Press 1943).
3. McCandless, Boyd, *Children and Adolescents* (New York: Holt, Reinehart and Winston, 1961), pp. 13-14.
4. Spock, Benjamin, M.D., *Baby and Child Care (Pocket Books/Simon & Schuster Inc, 1996)*
5. William Sears, M.D., & Martha Sears, R.N., *The Baby Book* (Boston: Little, Brown & Company, 1993), p. 343.
6. *Journal of Human Lactation*, Volume 14, Number 2, June 1998, p. 101.
7. Ibid., p. 101.

Chapter Three

1. This conclusion was drawn from a study based on 32 mother-infant pairs observed over two years. Sixteen families were from the La Leche League, and the other sixteen were not. "Sleep-Wake Patterns of Breast-Fed Infants in the First Two Years of Life," *Pediatrics* 77, no. 3, (March 1986): p. 328.
2. Marc Weissbluth, *Healthy Sleep Habits, Happy Child* (New York, Ballantine Books 1987), p. 44.
3. Ibid., p. 6.
4. American Academy of Pediatrics, "Does Bed Sharing Affect the Risk of SIDS?" *Pediatrics* 100, no. 2 (August 1997): p. 727.
5. American Academy of Pediatric Policy Statement, *Pedatrics*, Vol. 116 no. 5 November 2005, p. 1247.

Chapter Four

1. *Pediatrics,* 100, no. 6 (December 1997): p. 1035.
2. Ibid., p. 1036.
3. See www.cdc.gov/breastfeeding/data/reportcard.htm
4. See the work of Nancy Butte, Cathy Wills, Cynthia Jean, E. O'Brian Smith and Cutberto Garza, "Feeding Patterns of Exclusively Breastfed Infants During the First Four Months of Life," (Houston: USDA/ARS Children's Nutrition Research Center, 1985).
5. Sources supporting these recommended number of feeding times: *American Academy of Pediatrics Policy Statement Pediatrics* 100, no. 6, (December 1997): 1037; Frank Oski, M.D., *Principles and Practice of Pediatrics,* 2nd ed. (Philadelphia: J.B. Lippincott Company, 1994), p. 307; Richard E. Behrman, M.D., Victor C. Vaughan, M.D., Waldo E. Nelson, M.D., *Nelsons Textbook of Pediatrics*, 13th ed. (Philadelphia: W.B. Sauders Company, 1987), p. 124; Kathleen Huggins, *The Nursing Mother's Companion,* 3rd ed. (Boston: The Harvard Common Press, 1995), p. 35; Jan Riordan and Kathleen Auerbach, *Breastfeeding and Human Lactation,* (Sudbury, MA.: Jones and Bartlett Publishers,

1993), pp. 188, 189, 246.

6. Breastfeeding mothers are sometimes warned not to use a bottle. The concern is over "nipple confusion." The belief is that a baby will become confused and refuse the breast if offered a bottle. Although under normal circumstances there will be no need to introduce a bottle to the breast-fed infant in the first few weeks, there will come a time when the bottle will be a welcome friend. After the first few days of breastfeeding, supplementing by bottle rarely causes "nipple confusion." Kathleen Huggins, *The Nursing Mother's Companion,* 3rd ed. (Boston: Harvard Common Press, 1995), p. 73.

Chapter Seven

1. *Caring for Your Baby and Young Child—Birth to Age Five: The Complete and Authoritative Guide* (The American Academy of Pediatrics), ed. Steven P. Shelov M.D., F.A.A.P. (New York: Bantam Books, 1998), pp. 34-47.

2. Study cited by Mary Howell, M.D. in *baby!* Vol. 2 No.2. The Healthy Baby 1987, p. 27.

3. Ibid., p. 189.

4. Ibid., pp. 188-89.

5. Ibid., pp. 36.

Chapter Nine

1. Michael E. Lamb, Ph.D., from the Department of Pediatrics at the University of Utah Medical School, summarizes our position: "The preponderance of the evidence thus suggests that extended contact [the bonding theory] has no clear effects on maternal behavior." Michael E. Lamb, Ph.D., in *Pediatrics,* 70, no. 5 (November 1982), p. 768.

2. For an excellent challenge to the myth of bonding, please see Diane Eyer, *Mother Infant-Bonding: Scientific Fiction,* (New Haven: Yale University Press. 1992).

3. *Pediatrics* (August 1997), p. 272.

Subject Index

More Parenting Resources

With over eight million households worldwide to their credit, trusted parenting authors Pediatrician Robert Bucknam, and Gary Ezzo bring their collective wisdom, experience, and insights to bear on these critical phases of growth and development.

On Becoming Babywise II

This book provides the practical side of introducing solid foods, managing mealtimes, nap transitions, traveling with your infant, setting reasonable limits while encouraging healthy exploration and much more. Parents learn how to teach their baby basic sign language, a tool proven to help stimulate cognitive growth and advance communication.

On Becoming Pretoddlerwise

The period between 12 and 16 months places a child on a one-way bridge to the future. Infancy is a thing of the past and toddlerhood is straight ahead. A baby still? Not really, but neither is he a toddler, and that is the key to understanding this phase of growth. This is a period of metamorphosis when his potential for learning seems limitless, his budding curiosity unquenchable and his energy level never seems to diminish. It is also a period of great exchange: baby food is exchanged for table food; the highchair for booster seat; finger feeding is replaced with spoon; babbling sounds will transition to speaking; the first unsteady steps are conquered by strides of confidence, and the list goes on. *On Becoming Pretoddlerwise* will help any parent acquire useful knowledge that will prepare them for what lies around the next corner—the reality of toddlerhood where change sometimes comes every day.

On Becoming Toddlerwise

The toddler years are learning fields and you need a trustworthy guide to take you through the unfolding maze of your child's developing world. *On Becoming Toddlerwise* is a toolchest of workable strategies and ideas that multiply your child's learning opportunities in a loving and nurturing way. This resource is as practical as it is informative.

On Becoming Pottywise for Toddlers

Potty training does not have to be complicated and neither should a resource that explains it. *On Becoming Pottywise for Toddlers* looks to developmental readiness cues of children as the starting point of potty training. While no promise can be made we can tell you that many moms successfully complete their training in a day or two; some achieve it literally in hours.

On Becoming Preschoolwise

Gary Ezzo and Dr. Robert Bucknam once again bring their collective wisdom, experience, and insight to bear on this critical phase of preschool training. From teaching about the importance of play to learning how to prepare a preschooler for the first day of school, from organizing your child's week to understanding childhood fears and calming parental anxiety; sound advice and practical application await the reader.

On Becoming Childwise

Equip yourself with 15 practical principles for training kids in the art of living happily among family and friends. Foster the safe, secure growth of your child's self-concept and worldview. *On Becoming Childwise* shows you how to raise emotionally-balanced, intellectually-assertive and morally-sensible children. It is the essential guidebook for the adventurous years from toddler to grade-schooler!

On Becoming Preteenwise

The middle years, eight to twelve years of age, are perhaps the most significant attitude-forming period in the life of a child. It is during this time that the roots of moral character are established. From the foundation that is formed, healthy or not-so-healthy family relationships will be built. These are the years when patterns of behavior are firmly established—patterns that will impact your parent-child relationship for decades to come. Rightly meeting the small challenges of the middle years significantly reduces the likelihood of big challenges in the teen years.

On Becoming Teenwise

Why do teenagers rebel? Is it due to hormones, suppressed primal desires to stake out their own domain, or a natural and predictable process of growth? To what extent do parents encourage or discourage the storm and stress of adolescence? *On Becoming Teenwise* looks at the many factors that make living with a teenager a blessing or a curse. It exposes the notions of secular myth and brings to light the proven how-to applications of building and maintaining healthy relationships with your teens. Whether you worry about your teen and dating or your teen and drugs, the principles of *On Becoming Teenwise* are appropriate and applicable for both extremes and everyone in-between. They do work!